W9-AZQ-024

ECGs MADE EASY

POCKET REFERENCE

SECOND EDITION

Hazel Randall R.N

BARBARA AEHLERT, RN, BSPA
Southwest EMS Education, Inc.
Glendale, Arizona

Illustrations (except ECGs and those
otherwise noted) by Kimberly Battista

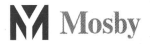 Mosby

An Imprint of Elsevier Science
St. Louis London Philadelphia Sydney Toronto

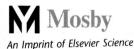

Mosby

An Imprint of Elsevier Science

Editor-in-Chief: *Andrew Allen*
Executive Editor: *Claire Merrick*
Developmental Editor: *Laura Bayless*
Project Manager: *John Rogers*
Senior Production Editor: *Helen Hudlin*
Designer: *Kathi Gosche*

Second EDITION

Copyright © 2002 by Mosby, Inc.

All rights reserved. No part of this publication may be reproduced or transmitted in any form or by any means, electronic or mechanical, including photocopy, recording, or any information storage and retrieval system, without permission in writing from the publisher.

NOTICE
Pharmacology is an ever-changing field. Standard safety precautions must be followed, but as new research and clinical experience broaden our knowledge, changes in treatment and drug therapy may become necessary or appropriate. Readers are advised to check the most current product information provided by the manufacturer of each drug to be administered to verify the recommended dose, the method and duration of administration, and contraindications. It is the responsibility of the licensed prescriber, relying on experience and knowledge of the patient, to determine dosages and the best treatment for each individual patient. Neither the publisher nor the editor assumes any liability for any injury and/or damage to persons or property arising from this publication.

Permission to photocopy or reproduce solely for internal or personal use is permitted for libraries or other users registered with the Copyright Clearance Center, provided that the base fee of $4.00 per chapter plus $.10 per page is paid directly to the Copyright Clearance Center, 222 Rosewood Drive, Danvers, Massachusetts 01923. This consent does not extend to other kinds of copying, such as copying for general distribution, for advertising or promotional purposes, for creating new collected works, or for resale.

Mosby, Inc.
An Imprint of Elsevier Science
11830 Westline Industrial Drive
St. Louis, Missouri 63146

Printed and bound in China

ISBN 0-323-01433-X

02   03   04   05   TG/RDC   9   8   7   6   5   4

PREFACE

The purpose of this pocket reference is to provide the health care provider with a handy, easy-to-use manual contaning the primary information needed to interpret basic cardiac dysrhythmias. ECG characteristics of each dysrhythmia are provided in table format for quick reference with possible patient signs and symptoms related to the dysrhythmia. Where appropriate, current recommended treatment for the dysrhythmia is discussed. All rhythm strips were recorded in lead II unless otherwise noted.

Features new to the second edition include:

- **Expanded anatomy and physiology and basic electrophysiology chapters.** Chapters 1 and 2 have been expanded to include a more in-depth discussion of the coronary blood supply, conduction system, waveforms, and lead placement.
- **12-lead ECG chapter.** A new chapter has been added providing an introduction to 12-lead ECG recognition. This chapter presents information including lead placement; bundle branch blocks; recognizing ECG signs of ischemia, injury, and infarction; chamber enlargement; and ECG changes associated with electrolyte disturbances.

Every attempt has been made to provide information that is consistent with current literature, including current resuscitation guidelines; however, the reader is advised to learn and follow local prototcols as defined by his/her medical advisors.

I hope you find this text of assistance and welcome your comments and suggestions.

Barbara Aehlert, RN

For my best friend,
Maryalice Witzel, RN
Thank you for always being there for me.

ACKNOWLEDGMENTS

I would like to thank:

- Patty Seneski, RN; Bill Loughran, RN; James Bratcher, CEP; Timothy Klatt, RN; Holly Button, CEP; Gretchen Chalmers, CEP; Thomas Cole, CEP; Brent Haines, CEP; Joe Martinez, CEP; Stephanos Orphanidis, CEP; Steve Ruehs, CEP; Dionne Socie, CEP; Kristina Tellez, CEP; and Fran Wojculewicz, RN, for providing many of the rhythm strips used in this text.
- Claire Merrick for her direction and support of this project. It is a pleasure working with you and your team.
- The Southwest EMS Education "team"—James Bratcher, CEP; Lynn Browne-Wagner, RN; Ken Bruck, CEP; Randy Budd, CEP; Thomas Cole, CEP; Bill Loughran, RN; Captain Garret Olson, CEP; Jeff Pennington, CEP; Captain Greg Ruiz, CEP; and Maryalice Witzel, RN, for the hours spent in the classroom and on the telephone discussing many topics that ultimately affect what we teach and how we deliver the information to our students.
- My family—Dean, Andrea, Sherri, Sean, and Tony. Thanks for your patience and taking care of things on a daily basis as I worked to complete this project.
- The reviewers of this text. Your thorough review, comments, and suggestions were sincerely appreciated. Areas of this text were rewritten, reorganized, and clarified because of your efforts. Thank you.

ABOUT THE AUTHOR

Barbara Aehlert, RN, is the President/CEO of Southwest EMS Education, Inc. in Arizona. She has been a registered nurse for more than 20 years with clinical experience in medical/surgical and critical care nursing and, for the past 15 years, in prehospital education. As an active instructor, Barbara regularly teaches courses related to the care of the adult cardiac patient and takes a special interest in teaching basic dysrhythmia recognition to nurses and paramedics.

In addition to this text and the accompanying *ECGs Made Easy*, Barbara is the author of the following Mosby publications: *ACLS Quick Review Study Guide*, *ACLS Quick Review Study Cards*, *ACLS Quick Review Slide Set*, *Mosby's ACLS Test Generator*, and *Pediatric Advanced Life Support Study Guide*. Barbara has also acted as a consultant on other Mosby educational materials, as a reviewer of several texts, and has contributed to several Mosby CD-ROM projects.

CONTENTS

CHAPTER 1

Anatomy and Physiology

LOCATION OF THE HEART

The heart is a hollow muscular organ that lies in the middle of the thoracic cavity **(mediastinum)** behind the sternum, between the lungs, and just above the diaphragm. It is surrounded by a protective sac (pericardium) and is attached to the thorax through the **great vessels** (pulmonary arteries and veins, aorta, superior and inferior vena cavae) (Figure 1-1).

The **apex** (bottom) of the heart is formed by the tip of the left ventricle. It is positioned just above the diaphragm to the left in an anterior position, at the fifth intercostal space, midclavicular line. The **base** (top) of the heart is at approximately the level of the second intercostal space. The anterior surface of the heart consists primarily of the right ventricle. The inferior (diaphragmatic) surface is formed by the right and left ventricles (predominantly the left) (Figure 1-2).

HEART CHAMBERS

The heart is divided into four chambers or cavities but functions as a two-sided pump. The two upper chambers are the right and left atria, and the two lower chambers are the right and left ventricles.

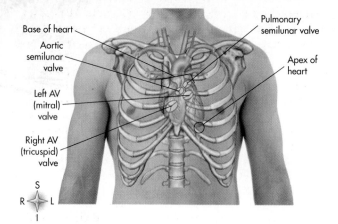

FIGURE 1-1 Location of the heart. Heart lies in the middle of the thoracic cavity (mediastinum) behind the sternum and between the lungs.

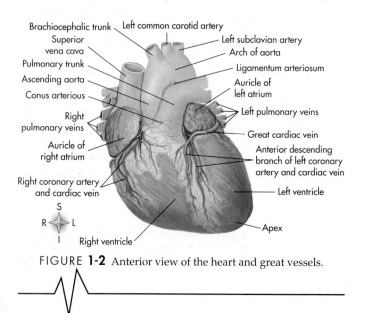

FIGURE 1-2 Anterior view of the heart and great vessels.

The right side of the heart is a low-pressure system that pumps venous blood to the lungs. The left side is a high-pressure system that pumps arterial blood to the systemic circulation.

The surface of the heart has grooves that indicate the positions of the **septa,** which separate the heart chambers. The coronary arteries and their major branches lie in these grooves. The septa are muscular partitions that separate the heart into two functional pumps: the right atrium and right ventricle (low-pressure pump), and the left atrium and left ventricle (high-pressure pump).

Atria

The **atria** are thin-walled, low-pressure chambers that *receive* blood. An internal wall of connective tissue called the *interatrial septum* separates the right and left atria. Externally, the coronary **sulcus** (groove) encircles the heart and separates the atria from the ventricles. It contains the coronary blood vessels and epicardial fat.

The right atrium receives deoxygenated blood from the superior vena cava (which carries blood from the head and upper extremities), the inferior vena cava (which carries blood from the lower body), and the coronary sinus (which receives blood from the intracardiac circulation). The left atrium receives oxygenated blood from the lungs via the right and left pulmonary veins.

There is normally a continuous flow of blood from the superior and inferior vena cavae into the atria. Approximately 70% of this blood flows directly through the atria and into the ventricles before the atria contract. With atrial contraction, an additional 30% is added to filling of the ventricles. This additional contribution of blood because of atrial contraction is called **atrial kick.**

Ventricles

The **ventricles** *pump* blood to the lungs and systemic circulation. An internal wall of connective tissue called the *interventricular septum* separates the right and left ventricles. Externally, the interventricular sulcus is anatomically divided into the anterior interventricular sulcus and the posterior interventricular sulcus. These grooves indicate the position of the interventricular septum (separating the right and left ventricles) and are perpendicular to the coronary sulcus (Figure 1-3).

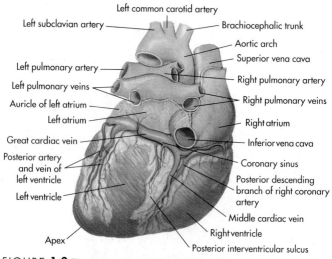

FIGURE **1-3** Posterior view of the heart and great vessels.

TABLE 1-1	LAYERS OF THE HEART WALL
Epicardium	External layer of the heart
	Coronary arteries, blood capillaries, lymph capillaries, nerve fibers, and fat are found in this layer
Myocardium	Middle and thickest layer of the heart
	Responsible for contraction of the heart
Endocardium	Innermost layer of the heart
	Lines the inside of the myocardium
	Covers the heart valves

The ventricles are larger and thicker-walled than the atria (Figure 1-4). The left ventricle is a high-pressure chamber that is approximately three times thicker than the right ventricle. To pump blood out of the left ventricle to the systemic circulation, it must contract forcefully and overcome arterial pressure and resistance. Each ventricle holds about 150 mL when full and normally ejects only about half this volume (70 to 80 mL) with each contraction.

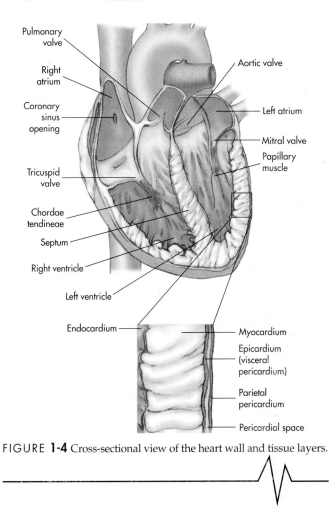

FIGURE **1-4** Cross-sectional view of the heart wall and tissue layers.

VALVES OF THE HEART

Atrioventricular (AV) Valves

The tricuspid valve is the AV valve that lies between the right atrium and right ventricle. It consists of three separate leaflets and is larger in diameter and thinner than the mitral valve. The mitral (or bicuspid) valve has only two cusps and lies between the left atrium and left ventricle.

Pressure within the atria rises as the atria fill with blood. This forces the tricuspid and mitral valves open (Figure 1-5) and allows deoxygenated blood to empty into the right ventricle and oxygenated blood to empty into the left ventricle. After the atria contract, the pressures in the atria and ventricles equalize and the tricuspid and mitral valves partially close. The ventricles then contract (systole), causing the pressure within the ventricles to rise sharply. The tricuspid and mitral valves close completely when the pressure within the ventricles exceeds that of the atria.

Semilunar (SL) Valves

The pulmonic and aortic valves are SL valves that prevent back-flow of blood from the aorta and pulmonary arteries into the ventricles during diastole (see Figure 1-5). Both sets of SL valves have three cusps shaped like half-moons.

The right ventricle ejects deoxygenated blood through the pulmonic valve into the right and left pulmonary arteries. The left ventricle ejects oxygenated blood through the aortic valve to the aorta, perfusing the body's organs and tissues.

During ventricular systole, the SL valves open, allowing blood to flow out of the ventricles. The SL valves close as systole ends and the pressure in the outflow arteries exceeds that of the ventricles.

The leaflets of the SL valves are smaller and thicker than the AV valves and do not have the support of chordae tendineae.

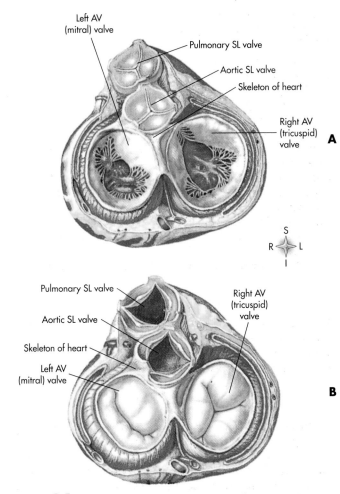

FIGURE 1-5 AV and semilunar valves. **A,** AV valves are open, semilunar valves are closed. **B,** AV valves are closed, semilunar valves are open.

The openings of the SL valves are smaller than the openings of the AV valves. As a result, the velocity of blood ejected through the aortic and pulmonary valves is much greater than that through the AV valves (Figure 1-6).

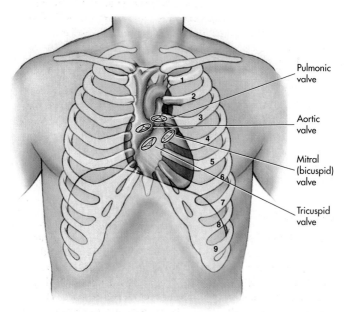

FIGURE **1-6** Anatomic location of heart valves.

Blood Flow Through the Heart

The right atrium receives blood low in oxygen and high in carbon dioxide from the superior and inferior vena cavae and the coronary sinus. Blood flows from the right atrium through the tricuspid valve into the right ventricle. When the right ventricle contracts, the tricuspid valve closes. The right ventricle expels the blood through the pulmonic valve into the pulmonary trunk. The pulmonary trunk divides into a right and left pulmonary artery, each of which carries blood to one lung (pulmonary circuit).

Blood flows through the pulmonary arteries to the lungs (where oxygen and carbon dioxide are exchanged in the pulmonary capillaries) and then to the pulmonary veins. Carbon dioxide is exhaled as the left atrium receives oxygenated blood from the lungs via the four pulmonary veins (two from the right lung and two from the left lung). Blood flows from the left atrium through the mitral (bicuspid) valve into the left ventricle. When the left ventricle contracts, the mitral valve closes. Blood leaves the left ventricle through the aortic valve to the aorta and its branches and is distributed throughout the body (systemic circuit). Blood from the tissues of the head and neck is emptied into the superior vena cava. Blood from the lower body is emptied into the inferior vena cava. The superior and inferior vena cavae carry their contents into the right atrium.

CARDIAC CYCLE

The cardiac cycle refers to a repetitive pumping process that includes all of the events associated with the flow of blood through the heart. The cycle has two phases for each heart chamber—systole and diastole. **Systole** is the period during which the chamber is contracting and blood is being ejected. Systole includes contraction of both atrial and ventricular muscle. **Diastole** is the period of relaxation during which the chamber is filling. Diastole includes relaxation of both atrial and ventricular muscle (Figure 1-7).

The cardiac cycle depends on the ability of the cardiac muscle to contract and the condition of the conduction system. The efficiency of the heart as a pump may be affected by abnormalities of cardiac muscle, the valves, or the conduction system.

During the cardiac cycle, the pressure within each chamber of the heart rises in systole and falls in diastole. The heart's valves

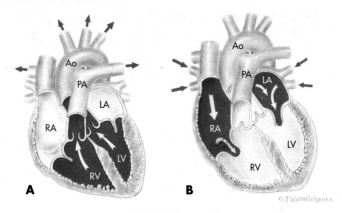

FIGURE **1-7** Blood flow during systole **(A)** and diastole **(B)**.

ensure that blood flows in the proper direction (Figure 1-8). Blood flows from one heart chamber to another if the pressure in the chamber is more than that in the next. These pressure relationships depend on the careful timing of contractions. The heart's conduction system provides the necessary timing of events between atrial and ventricular systole.

Heart Rate

The heart is innervated by both the sympathetic and parasympathetic divisions of the autonomic nervous system. The sympathetic division mobilizes the body, allowing the body to function under stress ("fight-or-flight" response). The parasympathetic division is responsible for the conservation and restoration of body resources ("feed-and-breed" response). Autonomic regulation of the cardiovascular system requires sensors, afferent pathways, an integration center, efferent pathways, and receptors.

Nerve impulses are carried from the sensory receptors to the brain by means of the vagus and glossopharyngeal nerves (afferent pathways). The medulla of the brain serves as the inte-

TABLE 1-2	CORONARY ARTERIES	
Coronary artery and its branches	**Portion of myocardium supplied**	**Portion of conduction system supplied**
RIGHT		
Posterior descending	Right atrium	SA node (50% to 60% of population)
Right marginal	Right ventricle Inferior wall of left ventricle Posterior wall of left ventricle Posterior third of interventricular septum	AV node (85% to 90%) Proximal portion of bundle of His Posterior-inferior fascicle of left bundle branch
LEFT		
Anterior descending	Anterior and part of lateral surface of left ventricle Anterior two thirds of interventricular septum	Majority of right bundle branch Anterior-superior fascicle of left bundle branch Portion of the posterior-inferior fascicle of the left bundle branch
Circumflex	Left atrium Anterolateral and posterolateral walls of left ventricle Posterior wall of left ventricle	SA node (40% to 50% of population) AV node (10% to 15% of population)

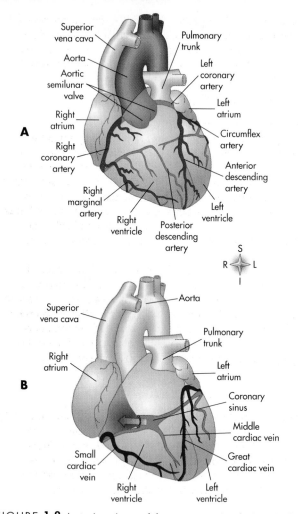

FIGURE 1-8 Anterior views of the coronary circulation. A, Coronary arteries. B, Coronary veins.

gration center and interprets the sensory information received. The medulla determines what body parameters need adjustment (if any) and transmits that information to the heart and blood vessels by means of motor nerves (efferent pathways).

Parasympathetic Stimulation

Parasympathetic Receptor Sites
Parasympathetic (inhibitory) nerve fibers supply the SA node, atrial muscle, and the AV junction of the heart by means of the vagus nerves. Acetylcholine, a neurotransmitter, is released when parasympathetic (cholinergic) nerve fibers are stimulated. Acetylcholine binds to parasympathetic receptors. The two main types of parasympathetic receptors are nicotinic and muscarinic receptors. Nicotinic receptors are located in skeletal muscle. Muscarinic receptors are located in smooth muscle.

Parasympathetic stimulation slows the rate of discharge of the SA node, slows conduction through the AV node, decreases the strength of atrial contraction, and can cause a small decrease in the force of ventricular contraction. (There is little effect on the strength of ventricular contraction because of minimal parasympathetic innervation of these chambers). The net effect of parasympathetic stimulation is slowing of the heart rate.

Sympathetic Stimulation

Sympathetic (accelerator) nerve fibers supply the sinoatrial (SA) node, atrioventricular (AV) node, atrial muscle, and the ventricular myocardium. Stimulation of sympathetic nerve fibers results in the release of norepinephrine, a neurotransmitter, which increases the force of ventricular contraction and the heart rate, blood pressure, and cardiac output (Figure 1-9).

Sympathetic Receptor Sites
Sympathetic (adrenergic) receptor sites are divided into alpha, beta, and dopaminergic receptors. Dopaminergic receptor sites are located in the coronary arteries and the renal, mesenteric,

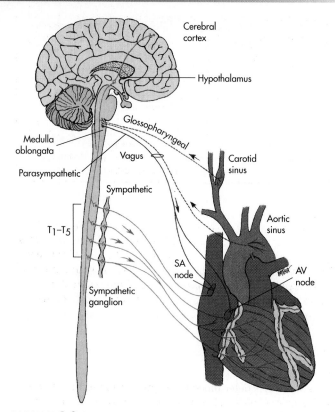

FIGURE 1-9 Autonomic nervous system innervation of the heart.

and visceral blood vessels. Stimulation of dopaminergic receptor sites results in dilation.

Different body tissues have different proportions of alpha and beta receptors. In general, alpha receptors are more sensitive to norepinephrine and beta receptors are more sensitive to epinephrine. Stimulation of alpha receptor sites results in constriction of blood vessels in the skin, cerebral, and **splanchnic** circulation.

TABLE 1-3	TERMINOLOGY
Chronotropic effect	Refers to a change in heart rate
	A positive chronotropic effect refers to an increase in heart rate
	A negative chronotropic effect refers to a decrease in heart rate
Inotropic effect	Refers to a change in myocardial contractility
	A positive inotropic effect results in an increase in myocardial contractility
	A negative inotropic effect results in a decrease in myocardial contractility

Beta-receptor sites are divided into beta-1 and beta-2. Beta-1 receptors are found in the heart. Stimulation of beta-1 receptors results in an increased heart rate, contractility, and, ultimately, irritability of cardiac cells. Beta-2 receptor sites are found in the lungs and skeletal muscle blood vessels. Stimulation of these receptor sites results in dilation of the smooth muscle of the bronchi and in blood vessel dilation.

Stroke Volume

Preload
Stroke volume is determined by the degree of ventricular filling during diastole **(preload)**, the pressure against which the ventricle must pump (afterload), and the myocardium's contractile state. Preload is the force exerted on the walls of the ventricles at the end of diastole. The volume of blood returning to the heart influences preload. More blood returning to the right atrium increases preload; less blood returning decreases preload.

Afterload
Afterload is the pressure or resistance against which the ventricles must pump to eject blood. Afterload is influenced by arterial blood pressure, arterial distensibility (ability to become

TABLE 1-4	REVIEW OF THE AUTONOMIC NERVOUS SYSTEM	
	Sympathetic division	Parasympathetic division
General effect	Fight-or-flight	Feed-and-breed
Primary neurotransmitter	Norepinephrine	Acetylcholine
EFFECTS OF STIMULATION		
Abdominal blood vessels	Constriction (alpha receptors)	No effect
Adrenal medulla	Increased secretion of epinephrine	No effect
Bronchioles	Dilation (beta receptors)	Constriction
Blood vessels of skin	Constriction (alpha receptors)	No effect
Blood vessels of skeletal muscle	Dilation (beta receptors)	No effect
Cardiac muscle	Increased rate and strength of contraction (beta receptors)	Decreased rate; decreased strength of atrial contraction, little effect on strength of ventricular contraction
Coronary blood vessels	Constriction (alpha receptors) Dilation (beta receptors)	Dilation

stretched), and arterial resistance. The less the resistance (lower afterload), the more easily blood can be ejected. Increased afterload (increased resistance) results in increased cardiac workload. Conditions that contribute to increased afterload include increased blood viscosity, hypertension, and aortic stenosis.

CHAPTER 2

Basic Electrophysiology

CARDIAC ACTION POTENTIAL

Cell membranes contain membrane channels. These channels are pores through which specific ions or other small, water-soluble molecules can cross the cell membrane from outside to inside (Figure 2-1). Permeability refers to the ability of a membrane channel to conduct ions once it is open.

A series of events causes the electrical charge inside the cell to change from its resting state (negative) to its depolarized (stimulated) state (positive) and back to its resting state (negative). The cardiac action potential is an illustration of these events in a single cardiac cell during polarization, depolarization, and repolarization. The stimulus that alters the gradient across the cell membrane may be electrical, mechanical, or chemical.

POLARIZATION, DEPOLARIZATION, AND REPOLARIZATION

Polarization

Polarization (also called the *resting membrane potential*) is the resting state during which no electrical activity occurs in the

17

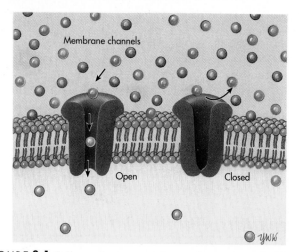

FIGURE **2-1** Cell membranes contain membrane channels. These channels are pores through which specific icons or other small, water-soluble molecules can cross the cell membranes from outside to inside.

TABLE **2-1**	Cardiac Cell Types		
Kinds of cardiac cells	**Where found**	**Primary function**	**Primary property**
Myocardial cells	Myocardium	Contraction and relaxation	Contractility
Pacemaker cells	Electrical conduction system	Generation and conduction of electrical impulses	Automaticity Conductivity

Modified from Huszar RJ: *Basic dysrhythmias: interpretation and management,* ed 2, St Louis, 1994, Mosby.

heart. When a cardiac muscle cell is polarized, the inside of the cell is more negative than the outside because of the numbers and types of ions found inside the cell. The primary intracellular ions include K+ and several negatively charged ions (anions). During the resting state, K+ ions leak out of the cell, leaving the negatively charged ions inside the cell. The result is a negative charge inside the cell (Figure 2-2).

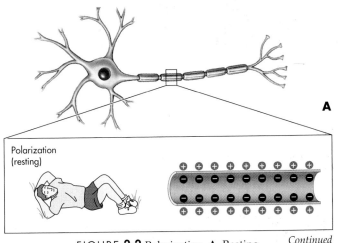

A

Polarization (resting)

FIGURE **2-2** Polarization. **A,** Resting.   *Continued*

Before the heart can mechanically contract and pump blood, cardiac muscle cell depolarization must take place. The terms *depolarization* and *repolarization* are used to describe the changes that occur in the heart when an impulse forms and spreads throughout the myocardium. Waveforms on the ECG correlate with depolarization and repolarization.

Depolarization

When the cardiac muscle cell is stimulated, the cell is said to depolarize (Figure 2-3). The inside of the cell becomes more

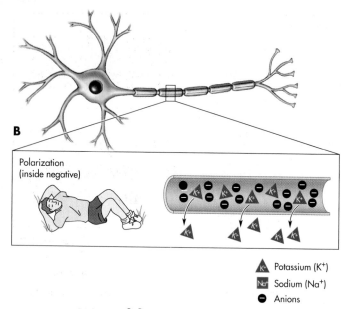

	Potassium (K⁺)
	Sodium (Na⁺)
	Anions

FIGURE **2-2**, cont'd **B,** Inside negative.

positive because of the entry of Na+ ions into the cell through Na+ membrane channels. Thus **depolarization** occurs because of the inward diffusion of Na+. Depolarization proceeds from the innermost layer of the heart (endocardium) to the outermost layer (epicardium). On the ECG, the P wave represents atrial depolarization, and the QRS complex represents ventricular depolarization.

Depolarization is **not** the same as contraction. Depolarization is an electrical event expected to result in contraction (a mechanical event). It is possible to view electrical activity on the cardiac monitor, yet evaluation of the patient reveals no palpable pulse. This clinical situation is termed *pulseless electrical activity (PEA).*

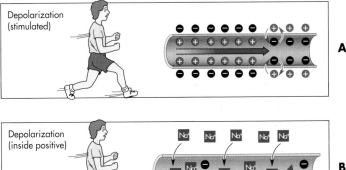

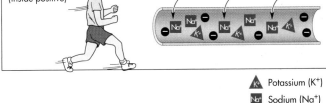

K⁺ Potassium (K⁺)
Na⁺ Sodium (Na⁺)
⊖ Anions

FIGURE **2-3** Depolarization. **A,** Stimulated. **B,** Inside positive.

Repolarization

After the cell depolarizes, the diffusion of Na+ into the cell stops. K+ is allowed to diffuse out of the cell, leaving the anions (negatively charged ions) inside the cell. Thus **repolarization** occurs because of the outward diffusion of K+. The membrane potential of the cell returns to its negative resting level (Figure 2-4). This causes the contractile proteins to separate (relax). The cell can then be stimulated again if another electrical impulse arrives at the cell membrane.

Repolarization proceeds from the epicardium to the endocardium. On the ECG, the ST segment represents early ventricular repolarization and the T wave represents ventricular repolarization.

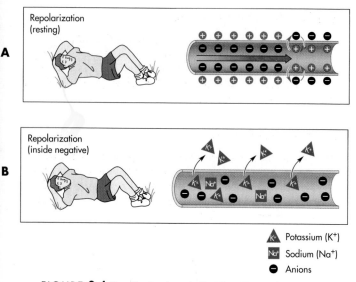

A

Repolarization
(resting)

B

Repolarization
(inside negative)

K⁺ Potassium (K⁺)
Na⁺ Sodium (Na⁺)
⊖ Anions

FIGURE **2-4** Repolarization. **A,** Resting. **B,** Inside negative.

REFRACTORY PERIODS

Refractoriness is a term used to describe the extent to which a cell is able to respond to a stimulus. In the heart, the refractory period is longer than the contraction itself.

Absolute Refractory Period

The *absolute* **refractory period** (also known as the *effective refractory period*) corresponds with the onset of the QRS complex to the peak of the T wave. During this period, the myocardial cell will not respond to further stimulation (the myocardial working cells cannot contract and the cells of the electrical conduction system cannot conduct an electrical impulse), no matter how strong the stimulus. Because of this mechanism, tetanic (sustained) contractions cannot be induced in cardiac muscle.

Relative Refractory Period

The *relative* **refractory period** (also known as the *vulnerable period*) corresponds with the downslope of the T wave. During this period, some cardiac cells have repolarized to their threshold potential and can be stimulated to respond (depolarize) to a stronger than normal stimulus.

Supernormal Period

After the relative refractory period is a **supernormal period** during which a weaker than normal stimulus can cause depolarization of cardiac cells. On the ECG, this corresponds with the end of the T wave. It is possible for cardiac dysrhythmias to develop during this period (Figure 2-5).

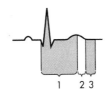

FIGURE **2-5** Absolute refractory period **(1)**, relative refractory period **(2)**, and the supernormal period **(3)**.

PROPERTIES OF CARDIAC CELLS

Cardiac cells have four primary characteristics:

- **Automaticity:** Ability of cardiac pacemaker cells to spontaneously initiate an electrical impulse without being stimulated from another source (such as a nerve). The SA node, AV junction, and Purkinje fibers normally possess this characteristic (Figures 2-6 and 2-7).
- **Excitability** (or **irritability**): A characteristic shared by all cardiac cells that refers to the ability of cardiac muscle cells, which are electrically irritable because of an ionic im-

balance across the membrane of the cells, to respond to an external stimulus, such as that from a chemical, mechanical, or electrical source.

- **Conductivity:** Ability of a cardiac cell to receive an electrical stimulus and conduct that impulse to an adjacent cardiac cell. All cardiac cells possess this characteristic. Intercalated disks present in the membranes of cardiac cells are responsible for the property of conductivity and allow an impulse in any part of the myocardium to spread throughout the heart. The speed of conduction can be altered by factors such as sympathetic and parasympathetic stimulation and medications.
- **Contractility:** Ability of cardiac cells to shorten, causing cardiac muscle contraction in response to an electrical stimulus. Contractility can be enhanced with certain medications, such as digitalis, dopamine, and epinephrine.

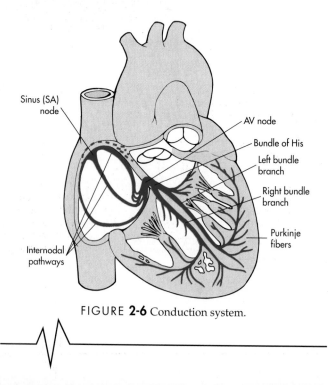

FIGURE **2-6** Conduction system.

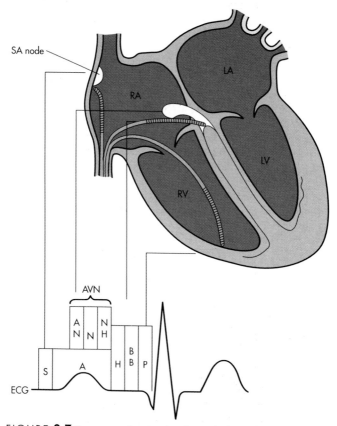

FIGURE **2-7** Sequence of activation through the conduction system. *S,* SA node conduction; *A,* atrial conduction; *AN,* atrionodal conduction; *N,* nodal conduction; *NH,* nodal–His conduction; *AVN,* AV nodal conduction; *H,* His bundle conduction; *BB,* bundle branch conduction; *P,* Purkinje fiber conduction; *RA,* right atrium; *LA,* left atrium; *RV,* right ventricle; *LV,* left ventricle.

TABLE 2-2   SUMMARY OF THE CONDUCTION SYSTEM

Structure	Location	Function
Sinoatrial node	Right atrial wall just inferior to opening of superior vena cava	Primary pacemaker; initiates impulse that is normally conducted throughout the left and right atria; intrinsic rate 60-100 beats/min
Atrioventricular node	Posterior septal wall of the right atrium immediately behind the tricuspid valve and near the opening of the coronary sinus	Receives impulse from SA node and delays relay of the impulse to the bundle of His, allowing time for the atria to empty their contents into the ventricles before the onset of ventricular contraction
Bundle of His	Superior portion of interventricular septum	Receives impulse from AV node and relays it to right and left bundle branches; intrinsic pacemaker ability of 40-60 beats/min
Right and left bundle branches	Interventricular septum	Receives impulse from bundle of His and relays it to Purkinje fibers in ventricular myocardium
Purkinje fibers	Ventricular myocardium	Receives impulse from bundle branches and relays it to ventricular myocardium; intrinsic pacemaker ability of 20-40 beats/min

THE ELECTROCARDIOGRAM

The electrocardiogram (ECG) records as specific waveforms and complexes the electrical activity of a large mass of atrial and ventricular cells. Think of the ECG as a voltmeter that records the electrical voltages (potentials) generated by depolarization of heart muscle. This electrical activity within the heart is visually recorded by means of electrodes connected by cables to an ECG machine.

ECG monitoring may be used to monitor a patient's heart rate, evaluate the effects of disease or injury on heart function, evaluate pacemaker function, evaluate the response to medications (e.g., antidysrhythmics), and/or to obtain a baseline recording before, during, and after a medical procedure.

The ECG *can* provide information about the orientation of the heart in the chest, conduction disturbances, electrical effects of medications and electrolytes, the mass of cardiac muscle, and the presence of ischemic damage. The ECG does *not* provide information about the mechanical (contractile) condition of the myocardium. The effectiveness of the heart's mechanical activity is evaluated by assessment of the patient's pulse and blood pressure.

Electrodes

Electrodes are applied at specific locations on the patient's chest wall and extremities in combinations of two, three, four, or five to view the heart's electrical activity from different angles and planes. One end of a monitoring cable is attached to the electrode and the other end to an ECG machine.

Leads

A **lead** is a record of electrical activity between two electrodes. Each lead records the *average* current flow at a specific time in a portion of the heart.

Leads allow viewing of the heart's electrical activity in two different planes: frontal (coronal) or horizontal (transverse). Frontal plane leads view the heart from the front of the body. Directions in the frontal plane are superior, inferior, right, and left. Horizontal plane leads view the heart as if the body were sliced in half horizontally. Directions in the horizontal plane are anterior, posterior, right, and left. A 12-lead ECG provides views of the heart in both the frontal and horizontal planes and views the surfaces of the left ventricle from 12 different angles.

There are three types of leads: standard limb leads, augmented leads, and precordial (chest) leads. Each lead has a negative (−) and positive (+) electrode (pole). Moving the lead selector on the ECG machine allows any of the electrodes to be made positive or negative.

Think of the positive electrode as an eye. The position of the positive electrode on the body determines the portion of the heart "seen" by each lead (Figure 2-8). Each lead senses the magnitude and direction of the electrical forces caused by the spread of waves of depolarization and repolarization throughout the heart.

If the wave of depolarization (electrical impulse) moves toward the *positive* electrode, the waveform recorded on ECG graph

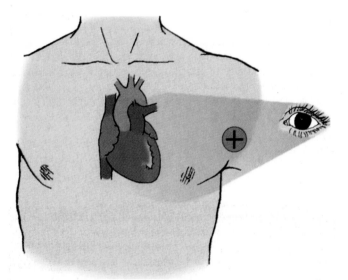

FIGURE **2-8** Each lead has a negative (−) and positive (+) electrode. The position of the positive electrode on the body determines the portion of the heart "seen" by each lead.

paper will be upright (positive deflection). If the wave of depolarization moves toward the *negative* electrode, the waveform recorded will be inverted (downward or negative deflection). A **biphasic** (partly positive, partly negative) waveform or a straight line is recorded when the wave of depolarization moves perpendicularly to the positive electrode (Figure 2-9).

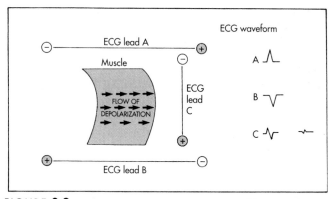

FIGURE **2-9 A,** If the wave of depolarization moves toward the positive electrode, the waveform recorded on the ECG graph paper will be upright. **B,** If the wave of depolarization moves toward the negative electrode, the waveform produced will be inverted. **C,** A biphasic (partly positive, partly negative) waveform is recorded when the wave of depolarization moves perpendicularly to the positive electrode.

TABLE 2-3	SUMMARY OF STANDARD LIMB LEADS		
Lead	Positive electrode	Negative electrode	Heart surface viewed
Lead I	Left arm	Right arm	Lateral
Lead II	Left leg	Right arm	Inferior
Lead III	Left leg	Left arm	Inferior

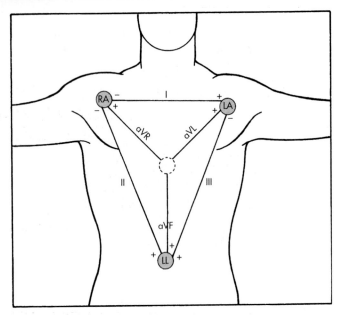

FIGURE **2-10** View of the standard limb leads and augmented leads.

Figures 2-10, 2-11, 2-12, and 2-13 show standard, augmented, modified, and precordial lead placement.

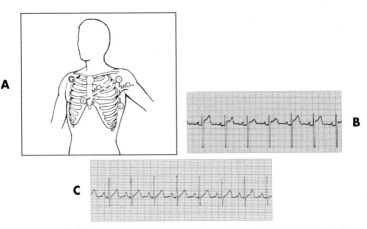

FIGURE **2-11** **A,** Electrode placement for MCL$_1$ and MCL$_6$. **B,** Typical ECG tracing MCL$_1$. **C,** Typical ECG tracing in MCL$_6$.

TABLE **2-4**	SUMMARY OF AUGMENTED LEADS	
Lead	Positive electrode	Heart surface viewed
Lead aVR	Right arm	None
Lead aVL	Left arm	Lateral
Lead aVF	Left leg	Inferior

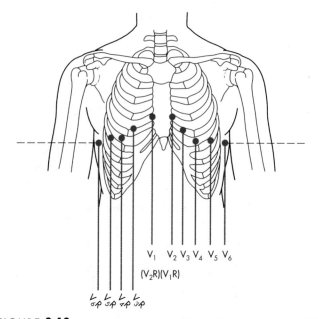

FIGURE **2-12** Anatomic placement of the left and right precordial leads.

TABLE **2-5**	SUMMARY OF PRECORDIAL LEADS	
Lead	Positive electrode position	Heart surface viewed
Lead V_1	Right side of sternum, fourth intercostal space	Septum
Lead V_2	Left side of sternum, fourth intercostal space	Septum
Lead V_3	Midway between V_2 and V_4	Anterior
Lead V_4	Left midclavicular line, fifth intercostal space	Anterior
Lead V_5	Left anterior axillary line at same level as V_4	Lateral
Lead V_6	Left midaxillary line at same level as V_4	Lateral

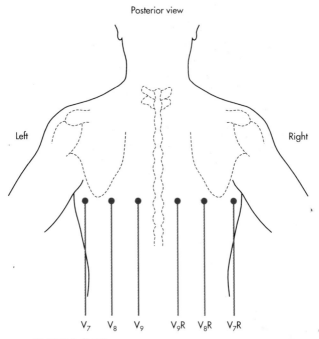

Posterior view

Left   Right

V₇   V₈   V₉   V₉R   V₈R   V₇R

FIGURE 2-13 Posterior precordial lead placement.

ECG PAPER

ECG paper is graph paper made up of small and large boxes.
The smallest boxes are 1-mm wide and 1-mm high. The horizontal axis of the paper corresponds with *time*. Time is stated in
seconds (Figure 2-14). ECG paper normally records at a constant
speed of 25 mm/sec. Thus each horizontal unit (1-mm box)
represents 0.04 sec (25 mm/sec $\times$ 0.04 sec = 1 mm). The lines
between every five small boxes on the paper are heavier and
indicate one large box. Because each large box is the width of
five small boxes, a large box represents 0.20 sec. Five large
boxes (each consisting of five small boxes) represent 1 second.

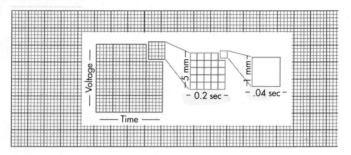

FIGURE **2-14** Horizontal axis represents time. Vertical axis represents amplitude or voltage.

Fifteen large boxes equal an interval of 3 seconds. Thirty large boxes represent 6 seconds.

The vertical axis of the graph paper represents *voltage* or *amplitude* of the ECG waveforms or deflections. Voltage may appear as a positive or negative value because voltage is a force with direction as well as amplitude.[1] The size or amplitude of a waveform is measured in millivolts (mV) or millimeters (mm).

The ECG machine's sensitivity must be calibrated so that a 1-mV electrical signal will produce a deflection measuring exactly 10-mm tall (Figure 2-15). When properly calibrated, a small box is 1-mm high (0.1 mV); a large box (equal to five small boxes) is

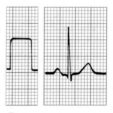

FIGURE **2-15** When the ECG machine is properly calibrated, a 1-mV electrical signal will produce a deflection measuring exactly 10-mm tall.

5-mm high (0.5 mV). Clinically, the height of a waveform is usually stated in millimeters not millivolts.

WAVEFORMS

A **waveform** or deflection is movement away from the baseline in either a positive (upward) or negative (downward) direction. A waveform that is partly positive and partly negative is *biphasic*. A waveform or deflection that rests on the baseline is *isoelectric*.

TABLE 2-6	TERMINOLOGY
Waveform	Movement away from the baseline in either a positive or negative direction
Segment	A line between waveforms; named by the waveform that precedes or follows it
Interval	A waveform and a segment
Complex	Several waveforms

P Wave

Electrical impulses originating in the SA node produce various waves on the ECG as they spread throughout the heart. The first wave in the cardiac cycle is called the *P wave*. The first half of the P wave is recorded when the electrical impulse that originated in the SA node stimulates the right atrium and reaches the AV node. The downslope of the P wave reflects stimulation of the left atrium. Thus the P wave represents atrial depolarization and the spread of the electrical impulse throughout the right and left atria. The atria contract a fraction of a second after the P wave begins. A waveform representing atria repolarization is usually not seen on the ECG because it is small and buried in the QRS complex.

The beginning of the P wave is recognized as the first abrupt or gradual deviation from the baseline, and its end is the point at which the waveform returns to the baseline (Figure 2-16).

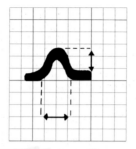

FIGURE **2-16** Normal P wave is usually no more than 2.5 mm in height and 0.11 sec in duration.

Normal Characteristics of the P Wave
- Smooth and rounded
- No more than 2.5 mm in height
- No more than 0.11 sec in duration (width)
- Positive in leads I, II, aVF, and V_2 through V_6
- May be positive, negative, or biphasic in leads III, aVL, and V_1

Abnormal P Waves
Tall and pointed (peaked) or wide and notched P waves may be seen in conditions such as chronic obstructive pulmonary disease (COPD), congestive heart failure (CHF), or valvular disease and may be indicative of atrial enlargement (Figure 2-17). Ectopic P waves may be either positive or negative in lead II. If the ectopic pacemaker is in the atria, the P wave will be upright; if the ectopic pacemaker is in the AV junction, the P wave will be negative (inverted) in lead II.

PR Segment

A **segment** is a line between waveforms and is named by the waveform that precedes or follows it. The *PR segment* is part of the PR interval and is the horizontal line between the end of the P wave and the beginning of the QRS complex. The PR segment is normally isoelectric. The His-Purkinje system is activated

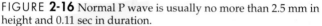

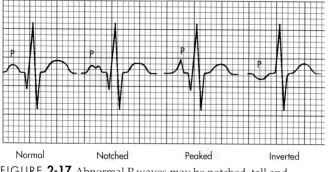

| Normal | Notched | Peaked | Inverted |

FIGURE **2-17** Abnormal P waves may be notched, tall and pointed (peaked), or inverted (negative).

during the PR segment. The duration of the PR segment depends on the duration of the P wave and impulse conduction through the AV junction.[2]

PR Interval

An **interval** is a waveform and a segment. The P wave plus the PR segment equals the *PR interval (PRI)* (Figure 2-18). The PR interval reflects depolarization of the right and left atria (P wave)

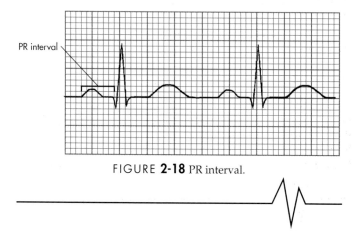

PR interval

FIGURE **2-18** PR interval.

and the spread of the impulse through the AV node, bundle of
His, right and left bundle branches, and the Purkinje fibers (PR
segment). The PR interval is measured from the point where the
P wave leaves the baseline to the beginning of the QRS complex.

Normal Characteristics of the PR Interval
- A normal PR interval indicates the electrical impulse was
  conducted normally through the atria, AV node, bundle of
  His, bundle branches, and Purkinje fibers
- Normally measures 0.12 to 0.20 sec in adults; may be shorter
  in children and longer in older persons
- Normally shortens as heart rate increases

Abnormal PR Intervals
A long PR interval (greater than 0.20 sec) indicates the impulse was
delayed as it passed through the atria or AV node. The P wave associated with a prolonged PR interval may be normal or abnormal.

A PR interval of **less** than 0.12 sec may be seen when the impulse
originates in an ectopic pacemaker in the atria close to the AV
node or in the AV junction. A shortened PR interval may also
occur if the electrical impulse progresses from the atria to the ventricles through an abnormal conduction pathway that bypasses
the AV node and depolarizes the ventricles earlier than usual.

QRS Complex

A **complex** consists of several waveforms. The *QRS complex*
consists of the Q wave, R wave, and S wave and represents the
spread of the electrical impulse through the ventricles (ventricular depolarization). Depolarization triggers contraction of ventricular tissue. Thus, shortly after the QRS complex begins, the
ventricles contract. The QRS complex is significantly larger than
the P wave because depolarization of the ventricles involves a
considerably greater muscle mass than depolarization of the
atria. A QRS complex normally follows each P wave. One or
even two of the three waveforms that make up the QRS complex may not always be present.

Variations of the QRS Complex
Although the term *QRS complex* is used, not every QRS complex contains a Q wave, R wave, and S wave. The Q wave is the first deflection of the QRS complex. A Q wave is *always* negative (below the baseline). The R wave is the first positive deflection (above the baseline) in the QRS complex. A negative deflection following the R wave is called an *S wave.*

If the QRS complex consists entirely of a positive waveform, it is called an *R wave.* If the complex consists entirely of a negative waveform, it is called a *QS wave.* If there are two positive deflections in the same complex, the second is called *R prime* and is written *R'*. If there are two negative deflections following an R wave, the second is written *S'*. Capital (upper case) letters are used to designate waveforms of relatively large amplitude and small (lower case) letters are used to label relatively small waveforms (Figure 2-19).

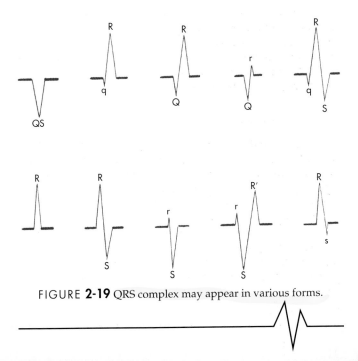

FIGURE **2-19** QRS complex may appear in various forms.

Measuring the Duration of the QRS Complex
The width of a QRS complex is most accurately determined when it is viewed and measured in more than one lead. The measurement should be taken from the QRS complex with the longest duration and clearest onset and end. The beginning of the QRS is measured from the point where the first wave of the complex begins to deviate from the baseline. The point at which the last wave of the complex begins to level out at, above, or below the baseline marks the end of the QRS complex.

Normal Characteristics of the QRS Complex
- The normal duration of the QRS complex in an adult varies between 0.06 and 0.10 sec
- With the exception of leads III and aVR, a normal Q wave is less than 0.04 sec in duration and less than 25% of the amplitude of the R wave in that lead
- QRS complex is predominantly positive in leads I, aVL, V_5, V_6 and in II, III, aVF; predominantly negative in leads aVR, V_1, V_2, and normally biphasic in leads V_3, V_4, and sometimes III

Abnormal QRS Complexes
- Duration of an abnormal QRS complex is greater than 0.10 sec
- Duration of a QRS complex caused by an electrical impulse originating in an ectopic pacemaker in the Purkinje network or ventricular myocardium is usually greater than 0.12 sec and often 0.16 sec or greater
- If the electrical impulse originates in a bundle branch, the duration of the QRS may be only slightly greater than 0.10 sec
- Enlargement of the right ventricle produces an abnormally prominent R wave; left ventricular enlargement produces an abnormally prominent S wave

ST Segment

The portion of the ECG tracing between the QRS complex and the T wave is known as the ST segment. The term *ST segment* is used regardless of whether the final wave of the QRS complex

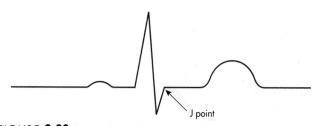

FIGURE **2-20** Point where the QRS complex and the ST segment meet is the *junction* or *J point*.

is an R or an S wave. The point where the QRS complex and the ST segment meet is called the *junction* or *J point* (Figure 2-20).

The ST segment represents the early part of repolarization of the right and left ventricles. The normal ST segment begins at the isoelectric line, extends from the end of the S wave, and curves gradually upward to the beginning of the T wave.

The PR segment is used as the baseline from which to evaluate the degree of displacement of the ST segment from the isoelectric line. To determine the degree of displacement, measure at a point 0.04 sec (one small box) after the J point. The ST segment is considered *elevated* if the segment is deviated above the baseline of the PR segment; it is considered *depressed* if the segment deviates below it. ST segment elevation or depression is considered "significant" if the displacement is more than 1 mm (one box) and is seen in two or more leads facing the same anatomic area of the heart.

Normal Characteristics of the ST Segment
- Begins with the end of the QRS complex and ends with the onset of the T wave
- In the limb leads, the normal ST segment is isoelectric (flat) but may normally be slightly elevated or depressed (usually by less than 1 mm)

- In some precordial leads, the ST segment may be normally elevated by as much as 2 to 3 mm; in the left precordial leads, ST segment elevation is not normally more than 1 mm

Abnormal ST Segments
- ST segment depression of more than 1 mm is suggestive of myocardial ischemia; ST segment elevation of more than 1 mm in the limb leads or 2 mm in the precordial leads is suggestive of myocardial injury
- A horizontal ST segment (forms a sharp angle with the T wave) is suggestive of ischemia
- Digitalis causes a depression (scoop) of the ST segment sometimes referred to as a "dig dip"

T Wave

Ventricular repolarization is represented on the ECG by the *T wave.* The absolute refractory period is still present during the beginning of the T wave. At the peak of the T wave, the relative refractory period has begun. It is during that period that a stronger than normal stimulus may produce ventricular dysrhythmias.

The normal T wave is slightly asymmetric where the peak of the waveform is closer to its end than the beginning, and the first half has a more gradual slope than the second half. The beginning of the T wave is identified as the point where the slope of the ST segment appears to become abruptly or gradually steeper. The T wave ends when it returns to the baseline. It may be difficult to clearly determine the onset and end of the T wave (Figure 2-21).

The T wave is normally oriented in the same direction as the preceding QRS complex. This is because epicardial cells repolarize earlier than endocardial cells. This causes the wave of repolarization to spread in the direction opposite depolarization. The result is a T wave deflected in the same direction as the QRS complex.[3]

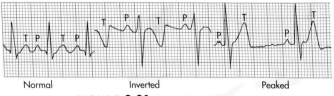

FIGURE **2-21** Examples of T waves.

Normal Characteristics of the T Wave
- Slightly asymmetric
- T wave is not normally more than 5 mm in height in any limb leads or 10 mm in any precordial lead; T waves are not normally less than 0.5 mm in height in leads I and II
- T waves are normally positive in leads I, II, V_2 to V_6; negative in lead aVR, positive in leads aVL and aVF, but may be negative if the QRS complex is less than 6 mm in height; and may be positive or negative in leads III and V_1

Abnormal T Waves
- T wave following an abnormal QRS complex is usually opposite in direction of the QRS
- Negative T waves suggest myocardial ischemia
- Tall, pointed (peaked) T waves are commonly seen in hyperkalemia
- Significant cerebral disease (e.g., subarachnoid hemorrhage) may be associated with deeply inverted T waves that are often called *cerebral T waves*

QT Interval

The QT interval represents total ventricular activity—the time from ventricular depolarization (activation) to repolarization (recovery). The term *QT interval* is used regardless of whether the QRS complex begins with a Q or R wave.

The QT interval is measured from the beginning of the QRS complex to the end of the T wave. In the absence of a Q wave, the QT interval is measured from the beginning of the R wave to the end of the T wave. The duration of the QT interval varies according to age, gender, and particularly heart rate. As the heart rate increases, the QT interval decreases. As the heart rate decreases, the QT interval increases.

To determine the duration of the QT interval, measure the interval between two consecutive R waves (R-R interval) and divide the number by two. Measure the QT interval. If the measured QT interval is less than half the R-R interval, it is probably normal (Figure 2-22). A QT interval that is approximately half the R-R interval is considered "borderline." A QT interval that is more than half the R-R interval is considered prolonged.

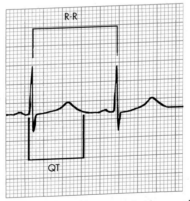

FIGURE **2-22** Measuring the QT interval. Abnormal QT interval prolongation in a patient taking quinidine.

U Wave

A *U wave* is a small waveform that, when seen, follows the T wave (Figure 2-23). The mechanism of the U wave is not definitely known. One theory suggests that it represents repolariza-

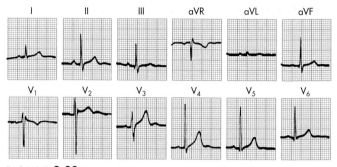

FIGURE **2-23** Normal U waves (best viewed in leads V_2 through V_4) in a 22-year-old male.

tion of the Purkinje fibers. U waves are most easily seen when the heart rate is slow and are difficult to identify when the rate exceeds 90 beats/min. When seen, U waves are normally tallest in leads V_2 and V_3.

Characteristics of the U Wave
- Rounded and symmetric
- Usually less than 2 mm in height and smaller than that of the preceding T wave
- In general, a U wave of more than 1.5 mm in height in any lead is considered abnormal

RATE MEASUREMENT

Method 1: Six-Second Method

Most ECG paper in use today is printed with 1-sec or 3-sec markers on the top or bottom of the paper. To determine the ventricular rate, count the number of *complete* QRS complexes within a period of 6 seconds and multiply that number by 10 to find the number of complexes in 1 minute. This method may be used for regular and irregular rhythms and is the simplest, quickest, and most commonly used method of rate measurement.

Method 2: Large Boxes

To determine the ventricular rate, count the number of large boxes between two consecutive R waves (R-R interval) and divide into 300. To determine the atrial rate, count the number of large boxes between two consecutive P waves (P-P interval) and divide into 300.

Table 2-7 illustrates heart rate determination using the large boxes method.

TABLE 2-7	HEART RATE DETERMINATION BASED ON THE NUMBER OF LARGE BOXES		
Number of large boxes	Heart rate (beats/min)	Number of large boxes	Heart rate (beats/min)
1	300	6	50
2	150	7	43
3	100	8	38
4	75	9	33
5	60	10	30

Method 3: Small Boxes

Each 1-mm box on the graph paper represents 0.04 sec. There are 1500 boxes in 1 minute (60 sec/minute divided by 0.04 sec/box = 1500 boxes/min). To calculate the ventricular rate, count the number of small boxes between two consecutive R waves and divide into 1500. To determine the atrial rate, count the number of small boxes between two consecutive P waves and divide into 1500.

Method 4: Sequence Method

To determine ventricular rate, select an R wave that falls on a dark vertical line. Number the next six consecutive dark vertical lines as follows: 300, 150, 100, 75, 60, and 50. Note where the next R wave falls in relation to the six dark vertical lines already marked. This is the heart rate.

RHYTHM/REGULARITY

The waveforms on an ECG strip are evaluated for regularity by measuring the distance between the P waves and QRS complexes. If the rhythm is regular, the R-R intervals (or P-P intervals if assessing atrial rhythm) are the same. Generally, a variation of plus or minus 10% is acceptable. For example, if there are 10 small boxes in an R-R interval, an R wave could be "off" by 1 small box and still be considered regular.

Ventricular Rhythm

To evaluate the regularity of the ventricular rhythm, measure the distance between two consecutive R-R intervals. Place one point of a pair of calipers (or make a mark on a piece of paper) on the beginning of an R wave. Place the other point of the calipers (or make a second mark on the paper) on the beginning of the R wave of the next QRS complex. Without adjusting the calipers, evaluate each succeeding R-R interval. (If paper is used, lift the paper and move it across the rhythm strip). Compare the distance measured with the other R-R intervals. If the ventricular rhythm is regular, the R-R intervals will measure the same.

Atrial Rhythm

To determine if the atrial rhythm is regular or irregular, follow the same procedure previously described for evaluation of ventricular rhythm but measure the distance between two consecutive P-P intervals (instead of R-R intervals) and compare that distance with the other P-P intervals. The P-P intervals will measure the same if the atrial rhythm is regular.

ANALYZING A RHYTHM STRIP

A methodical approach should be used when analyzing a rhythm strip to ensure accurate interpretation. Begin analyzing the rhythm strip from left to right.

Assess the Rate

To determine the ventricular rate, measure the distance between two consecutive R waves (R-R interval). To determine the atrial rate, measure the distance between two consecutive P waves (P-P interval). A **tachycardia** exists if the rate is more than 100 beats/ min. A **bradycardia** exists if the rate is less than 60 beats/min.

Assess Rhythm/Regularity

To determine if the ventricular rhythm is regular or irregular, measure the distance between two consecutive R-R intervals and compare that distance with the other R-R intervals. If the ventricular rhythm is regular, the R-R intervals will measure the same.

To determine if the atrial rhythm is regular or irregular, measure the distance between two consecutive P-P intervals and compare that distance with the other P-P intervals. If the atrial rhythm is regular, the P-P intervals will measure the same.

Identify and Examine P Waves

To locate P waves, look to the left of each QRS complex. Normally, one P wave precedes each QRS complex; they occur regularly and appear similar in size, shape, and position. If no P wave is present, the rhythm originated in the AV junction or the ventricles.

If one P wave is present before each QRS and the QRS is **narrow:**

- Is the P wave positive? If so, the rhythm probably originated from the SA node.
- Is the P wave negative or absent? If so, and the QRS complexes occur regularly, the rhythm probably originated from the AV junction.

Assess Intervals (Evaluate Conduction)

PR Interval (PRI)

Measure the PR interval. The PR interval is measured from the point where the P wave leaves the baseline to the beginning of the QRS complex. The normal PR interval is 0.12 to 0.20 sec. If the PR intervals are the same, they are said to be constant. If the PR intervals are different, is there a pattern? In some dysrhythmias, the duration of the PR interval will increase until a P wave appears with no QRS after it. This is referred to as *lengthening* of the PR interval. PR intervals that vary in duration and have no pattern are said to be *variable.*

QRS Duration

Identify the QRS complexes and measure their duration. The beginning of the QRS is measured from the point where the first wave of the complex begins to deviate from the baseline. The point at which the last wave of the complex begins to level out at, above, or below the baseline marks the end of the QRS complex. A QRS complex is narrow (normal) if it measures 0.10 sec or less and wide if it measures more than 0.10 sec.

QT Interval

Measure the QT interval in the leads that show the largest amplitude T waves. The QT interval is measured from the beginning of the QRS complex to the end of the T wave. In the absence of a Q wave, the QT interval is measured from the beginning of the R wave to the end of the T wave. If the measured QT interval is less than half the R-R interval, it is probably normal. This method of

QT interval measurement works well as a general guideline until the ventricular rate exceeds 100 beats/min.

Evaluate the Overall Appearance of the Rhythm

ST Segment
The ST segment is usually isoelectric in the limb leads. ST segment elevation or depression is determined by measuring at a point 0.04 sec (one small box) after the end of the QRS complex. The PR segment is used as the baseline from which to evaluate the degree of displacement of the ST segment from the isoelectric line (elevation or depression).

The ST segment is considered *elevated* if the segment is deviated above the baseline of the PR segment and *depressed* if the segment deviates below it. ST segment elevation or depression is considered "significant" if the displacement is more than 1 mm (one box) and is seen in two or more leads facing the same anatomic area of the heart.

T Wave
Evaluate the T waves. Are the T waves upright and of normal height? The T wave following an abnormal QRS complex is usually opposite in direction of the QRS. Negative T waves suggest myocardial ischemia. Tall, pointed (peaked) T waves are commonly seen in hyperkalemia.

Interpret the Rhythm and Evaluate Its Clinical Significance

Interpret the rhythm, specifying its site of origin (pacemaker site) (sinus), the mechanism (bradycardia), and the ventricular rate. For example, "sinus bradycardia at 38 beats/min." Evaluate the patient's clinical presentation to determine how he or she is tolerating the rate and rhythm.

ECG WAVEFORMS AND INTERVALS

Figure 2-24 displays the ECG waveforms, and Figure 2-25 displays the principal ECG segments and intervals.

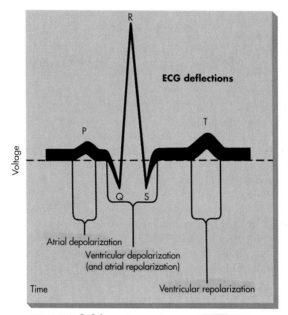

FIGURE **2-24** ECG waveforms: P, QRS, and T.

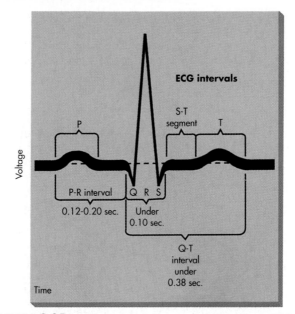

FIGURE **2-25** ECG segments and intervals: PR interval, QRS duration, ST segment, QT interval.

ARTIFACT

Accurate ECG rhythm recognition requires a tracing free from distortion or **artifact.** Artifact can be caused by many factors (Figures 2-26, 2-27, 2-28).

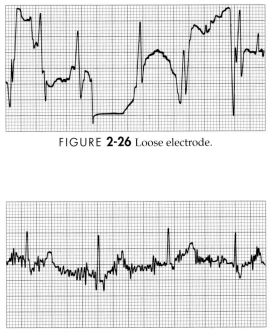

FIGURE **2-26** Loose electrode.

FIGURE **2-27** Artifact caused by muscle tremors.

FIGURE **2-28** 60-cycle interference.

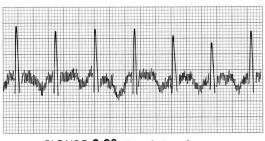

CHAPTER 3

Sinus Mechanisms

The normal heartbeat is the result of an electrical impulse that originates in the sinoatrial (SA) node. Normally, pacemaker cells within the SA node spontaneously depolarize more rapidly than other cardiac cells, thus dominating other areas that may be depolarizing at a slightly slower rate. The impulse is then transmitted to transitional cells at the periphery of the SA node and subsequently to the myocardial cells of the surrounding atrium. A rhythm originating from the SA node will have one positive (upright) P wave before each QRS complex.

SINUS RHYTHM

The SA node normally initiates electrical impulses at a rate of 60 to 100 beats/min. This rate is faster than any other part of the conduction system. As a result, the SA node is normally the primary pacemaker of the heart. **Sinus rhythm** is the name given a rhythm reflecting normal electrical activity—that is, the rhythm originates in the SA node and follows the normal pathway of conduction through the atria, AV junction, bundle branches, and ventricles, resulting in atrial and ventricular depolarization (Figure 3-1 and Table 3-1).

TABLE **3-1**	CHARACTERISTICS OF SINUS RHYTHM
Rate	60-100 beats/min
Rhythm	Regular
P waves	Uniform in appearance, positive (upright) in lead II, one precedes each QRS complex
PR interval	0.12-0.20 sec and constant from beat to beat
QRS duration	0.10 sec or less

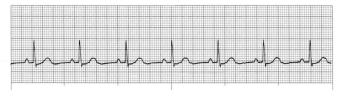

FIGURE **3-1** Sinus rhythm at 70 beats/min.

SINUS BRADYCARDIA

TABLE **3-2**	CHARACTERISTICS OF SINUS BRADYCARDIA
Rate	Less than 60 beats/min
Rhythm	Regular
P waves	Uniform in appearance, positive (upright) in lead II, one precedes each QRS complex
PR interval	0.12-0.20 sec and constant from beat to beat
QRS duration	0.10 sec or less

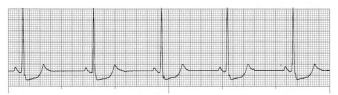

FIGURE **3-2** Sinus bradycardia at 48 beats/min; ST depression.

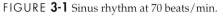

Causes and Clinical Significance

Sinus bradycardia (Figure 3-2 and Table 3-2) may be normal in physically conditioned adults and during sleep. However, it is the most common dysrhythmia associated with acute myocardial infarction,[4] often seen in patients with inferior and posterior infarction.

Other causes of sinus bradycardia include disease of the SA node, increased vagal (parasympathetic) tone (vomiting, increased intracranial pressure, vagal maneuvers, carotid sinus pressure), hypoxia, hypothermia, anorexia nervosa, hypothyroidism, hyperkalemia, uremia, glaucoma, sleep apnea syndrome, and administration of medications such as calcium channel blockers (verapamil, diltiazem), digitalis, and beta-blockers (propranolol).

Remember that cardiac output = stroke volume × heart rate. Therefore a decrease in either stroke volume *or* heart rate may result in a decrease in cardiac output.

Decreasing cardiac output will eventually produce myocardial ischemia and further hemodynamic compromise. Clinical signs and symptoms of hemodynamic compromise include hypotension, chest pain, shortness of breath, changes in mental status, left ventricular failure, a fall in urine output, and cold, clammy skin.

Intervention

No intervention is necessary if the patient is asymptomatic. If the patient is symptomatic because of the bradycardia, interventions may include oxygen, IV access, and administration of atropine and/or transcutaneous pacing.

SINUS TACHYCARDIA

TABLE **3-3**	CHARACTERISTICS OF SINUS TACHYCARDIA
Rate	101-180 beats/min
Rhythm	Regular
P waves	Uniform in appearance, positive (upright) in lead II, one precedes each QRS complex; at very fast rates it may be difficult to distinguish a P wave from a T wave
PR interval	0.12-0.20 sec and constant from beat to beat
QRS duration	0.10 sec or less

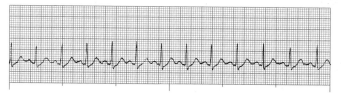

FIGURE **3-3** Sinus tachycardia at 129 beats/min.

Causes and Clinical Significance

Sinus tachycardia (Figure 3-3 and Table 3-3) occurs as a normal response to the body's demand for increased oxygen because of fever, pain and anxiety, hypoxia, congestive heart failure, acute myocardial infarction, infection, sympathetic stimulation, shock, hypovolemia, dehydration, exercise, and fright. Sinus tachycardia may also occur as the result of administration of medications such as epinephrine, atropine, dopamine, and dobutamine or substances such as caffeine-containing beverages, nicotine, and cocaine.

Sinus tachycardia is seen in about a third of patients with acute myocardial infarction,[2] especially those with an anterior infarction.[5] In the setting of acute MI, sinus tachycardia is a warning signal for heart failure, hypovolemia, and increased risk for serious dysrhythmias.

Intervention

Interventions are directed at correcting the underlying cause—i.e., fluid replacement, relief of pain, removal of offending medications or substances, reducing fever, and/or anxiety. Sinus tachycardia in a patient with an acute MI may be treated with beta-blockers. Beta-blockers are administered to slow the heart rate and decrease myocardial oxygen demand, provided there are no signs of heart failure or other contraindications to beta-blocker therapy.

SINUS ARRHYTHMIA

TABLE 3-4	CHARACTERISTICS OF SINUS ARRHYTHMIA
Rate	Usually 60-100 beats/min but may be slower or faster
Rhythm	Irregular, phasic with respiration; heart rate increases gradually during inspiration (R-R intervals shorten) and decreases with expiration (R-R intervals lengthen)
P waves	Uniform in appearance, positive (upright) in lead II, one precedes each QRS complex
PR interval	0.12-0.20 sec and constant from beat to beat
QRS duration	0.10 sec or less

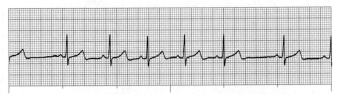

FIGURE 3-4 Sinus arrhythmia at 54 to 88 beats/min.

Causes and Clinical Significance

Respiratory sinus arrhythmia (Figure 3-4 and Table 3-4) is a normal phenomenon that occurs with respiration and changes in intrathoracic pressure. The heart rate increases with inspiration (R-R intervals shorten) and decreases with expiration (R-R intervals lengthen). Sinus arrhythmia is most commonly observed in infants and children but may be seen in any age group.

Nonrespiratory sinus arrhythmia is more likely seen in older individuals and in those with heart disease. It is common after acute inferior wall MI and may be seen with increased intracranial pressure. Nonrespiratory sinus arrhythmia may be the result of the effects of medications such as digitalis and morphine and carotid sinus pressure.[2]

Intervention

Sinus arrhythmia does not usually require intervention unless it is accompanied by a bradycardia that causes hemodynamic compromise. If hemodynamic compromise is present, IV atropine may be indicated.

SINOATRIAL (SA) BLOCK

TABLE 3-5	CHARACTERISTICS OF SINOATRIAL (SA) BLOCK
Rate	Usually normal but varies because of the pause
Rhythm	Irregular because of the pause(s) caused by the SA block—the pause is the same as (or an exact multiple of) the distance between two other P-P intervals
P waves	Uniform in appearance, positive (upright) in lead II; when present, one precedes each QRS complex
PR interval	0.12-0.20 sec and constant from beat to beat
QRS duration	0.10 sec or less

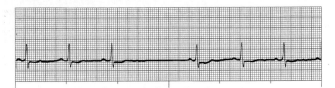

FIGURE **3-5** Sinoatrial (SA) block.

Causes and Clinical Significance

SA block (Figure 3-5 and Table 3-5) is relatively uncommon but may occur because of acute MI; digitalis, quinidine, procain-amide, or salicylate administration; coronary artery disease; myocarditis; congestive heart failure; carotid sinus sensitivity, or increased vagal tone.

If the episodes of SA block are frequent and/or accompanied by a slow rate, the patient may show signs and symptoms of hemodynamic compromise. Clinical signs and symptoms of hemodynamic compromise include hypotension, chest pain, shortness of breath, changes in mental status, left ventricular failure, a fall in urine output, and cold, clammy skin.

Intervention

If the episodes of SA block are transient and there are no signifi-cant signs or symptoms, the patient is observed. If signs of hemodynamic compromise are present and result from medica-tion toxicity, the offending agents should be withheld. If the episodes of SA block are frequent, IV atropine, temporary pac-ing, or insertion of a permanent pacemaker may be warranted.

SINUS ARREST

Causes and Clinical Significance

Causes of sinus arrest (Figure 3-6 and Table 3-6) include hypoxia,

TABLE 3-6	CHARACTERISTICS OF SINUS ARREST
Rate	Usually normal but varies because of the pause
Rhythm	Irregular—the pause is of undetermined length (more than one PQRST complex is omitted) and is not the same distance as other P-P intervals
P waves	Uniform in appearance, positive (upright) in lead II; when present, one precedes each QRS complex
PR interval	0.12-0.20 sec and constant from beat to beat
QRS duration	0.10 sec or less

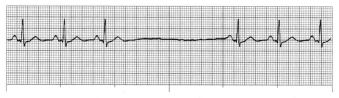

FIGURE 3-6 Sinus arrest.

myocardial ischemia or infarction, hyperkalemia, digitalis toxicity, reactions to medications such as beta-blockers and calcium channel blockers, carotid sinus sensitivity, or increased vagal tone. Signs of hemodynamic compromise such as weakness, lightheadedness, dizziness, or syncope may be associated with this dysrhythmia.

Intervention

If the episodes of sinus arrest are transient and there are no significant signs or symptoms, the patient is observed. If hemodynamic compromise is present, IV atropine may be indicated. If the episodes of sinus arrest are frequent and/or prolonged (more than 3 seconds), temporary pacing or insertion of a permanent pacemaker may be warranted.

CHAPTER 4

Atrial Rhythms

P waves reflect atrial depolarization. A rhythm originating from the SA node has one positive (upright) P wave before each QRS complex. A rhythm originating from the atria will have a positive P wave that is shaped differently than SA node–initiated P waves. This difference in P wave configuration occurs because the impulse originates in the atria and follows a different conduction pathway to the AV node.

PREMATURE ATRIAL COMPLEXES (PACS)

Premature beats may be produced by the atria, AV junction, or the ventricles. Premature beats appear *early*, that is, they occur before the next expected beat.

Premature beats are identified by their site of origin (atrial, junctional, or ventricular). A **premature atrial complex (PAC)** occurs when an irritable site (focus) within the atria discharges before the next SA node impulse is due to discharge, thus interrupting the sinus rhythm. If the irritable site is close to the SA node, the atrial P wave will look very similar to the P waves initiated by the SA node. The P wave of a PAC may be biphasic (partly positive, partly negative), flattened, notched, or pointed.

When compared with the P-P intervals of the underlying rhythm, a PAC is premature—occurring before the next expected sinus P wave (Figure 4-1 and Table 4-1). Premature atrial complexes are identified by:

- Early (premature) P waves
- Positive (upright) P waves (in lead II) that differ in shape from sinus P waves
- Early P waves that may or may not be followed by a QRS complex

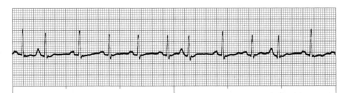

FIGURE **4-1** Sinus tachycardia with three PACs. *From the left,* beats 2, 7, and 10 are PACs.

TABLE **4-1**	CHARACTERISTICS OF PREMATURE ATRIAL COMPLEXES (PACS)
Rate	Usually within normal range but depends on underlying rhythm
Rhythm	Regular with premature beats
P waves	Premature (occurring earlier than the next expected sinus P wave), positive (upright) in lead II, one precedes each QRS complex, often differ in shape from sinus P waves—may be flattened, notched, pointed, biphasic, or lost in the preceding T wave
PR interval	May be normal or prolonged depending on the prematurity of the beat
QRS duration	Usually less than 0.10 sec but may be wide (aberrant) or absent, depending on the prematurity of the beat; the QRS of the PAC is similar in shape to those of the underlying rhythm unless the PAC is abnormally conducted

The PR interval of the PAC may be normal or prolonged, depending on the prematurity of the beat. QRS complexes associated with a PAC are typically identical or similar in shape and duration to those of the underlying rhythm because the impulse is conducted normally through the AV junction, bundle branches, and ventricles.

Aberrantly Conducted PACs

If a PAC occurs very early, the right bundle branch can be particularly slow to respond to the impulse *(refractory)*. The impulse travels down the left bundle branch without difficulty. Stimulation of the left bundle branch subsequently results in stimulation of the right bundle branch. Because of this delay in ventricular depolarization, the QRS will appear wide (greater than 0.10 sec). PACs associated with a wide QRS complex are called **aberrantly conducted PACs,** indicating conduction through the ventricles is abnormal (Figure 4-2).

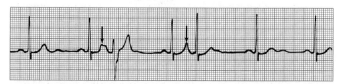

FIGURE **4-2** Premature atrial complexes with and without abnormal conduction (aberrancy). The first PAC *(arrow)* was conducted abnormally, producing a wide QRS complex. The second PAC *(arrow)* was conducted normally. Compare the T waves preceding each PAC with those of the underlying sinus bradycardia.

Noncompensatory vs. Compensatory Pause

A **noncompensatory (incomplete) pause** often follows a PAC and represents the delay during which the SA node resets its rhythm for the next beat. A **compensatory (complete) pause** often follows premature ventricular complexes (PVCs) (Box 4-1).

BOX **4-1**	DETERMINING COMPENSATORY VS. COMPENSATORY PAUSES

To determine whether or not the pause following a premature complex is compensatory or noncompensatory, measure the distance between three normal beats. Then compare that measurement to the distance between three beats, one of which includes the premature complex.

The pause is termed **noncompensatory** (or **incomplete**) if the normal beat following the premature complex occurs before it was expected (i.e., the period between the complex before and after the premature beat is less than two normal R-R intervals).

The pause is termed **compensatory** (or **complete**) if the normal beat following the premature complex occurs when expected (i.e., the period between the complex before and after the premature beat is the same as two normal R-R intervals).

Nonconducted PACs

Sometimes, when the PAC occurs very prematurely and close to the T wave of the preceding beat, only a P wave may be seen with no QRS after it (appearing as a pause) (Figure 4-3). This type of PAC is termed *nonconducted* or *blocked* PAC because the P wave occurred too early to be conducted. Nonconducted PACs occur because the AV junction is still refractory to stimulation and unable to conduct the impulse to the ventricles (thus no QRS complex).

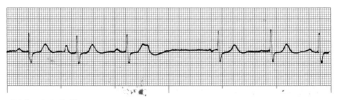

FIGURE **4-3** Sinus rhythm with a nonconducted (blocked) PAC.

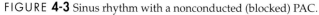

Causes and Clinical Significance

PACs are very common. Their presence does not necessarily imply underlying cardiac disease. PACs may occur because of emotional stress, congestive heart failure, myocardial ischemia or injury, mental and physical fatigue, atrial enlargement, digitalis toxicity, hypokalemia, hypomagnesemia, hyperthyroidism, and excessive intake of caffeine, tobacco, or alcohol. PACs may be present in up to half of all patients with acute myocardial infarction.[5]

The patient may complain of a "skipped beat" or occasional "palpitations" (if PACs are frequent) or may be unaware of their occurrence. Because the rhythm is irregular, count the patient's pulse for a full minute.

Intervention

PACs usually do not require treatment if they are infrequent; however, frequent PACs may initiate episodes of atrial fibrillation, atrial flutter, or paroxysmal supraventricular (atrial) tachycardia (PSVT). Frequent PACs are treated by correcting the underlying cause: reducing stress, reducing consumption of caffeine-containing beverages, treating congestive heart failure, or correcting electrolyte imbalances. If needed, frequent PACs may be treated with beta-blockers, calcium channel blockers, and/or antianxiety medications.

WANDERING ATRIAL PACEMAKER

Multiformed atrial rhythm is an updated term for the rhythm formerly known as **wandering atrial pacemaker.** With this rhythm, the size, shape, and direction of the P waves vary, sometimes from beat to beat. The differences in P wave configuration reflect gradual shifting of the dominant pacemaker between the SA node, the atria, and/or the AV junction (Figure 4-4). At least three different P wave configurations, seen in the same lead, are required for a diagnosis of wandering atrial pacemaker.

Lead II (continuous)

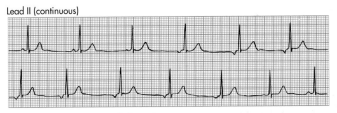

FIGURE **4-4** Wandering atrial pacemaker.

Wandering atrial pacemaker is associated with a normal or slow rate and irregular P-P, R-R, and PR intervals because of the different sites of impulse formation. The QRS duration is normally less than 0.10 sec because conduction through the ventricles is usually normal.

Causes and Clinical Significance

Wandering atrial pacemaker may be observed in normal, healthy hearts (particularly in athletes) and during sleep. It may also occur with some types of organic heart disease and with digitalis toxicity. This dysrhythmia usually produces no signs and symptoms unless it is associated with a bradycardic rate.

Interventions

If the rhythm occurs because of digitalis toxicity, the drug should be withheld.

MULTIFOCAL ATRIAL TACHYCARDIA

When the wandering atrial pacemaker is associated with a ventricular response of 100 beats/min or greater, the rhythm is termed **multifocal atrial tachycardia (MAT)** (Figure 4-5 and Table 4-2). MAT is also called *chaotic atrial tachycardia*. In MAT, multiple ectopic sites stimulate the atria. Multifocal atrial tachycardia may be confused with atrial fibrillation because both rhythms are irregular; however, P waves (although varying in size, shape, and direction) are clearly visible in MAT.

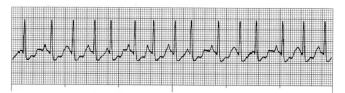

FIGURE **4-5** Multifocal atrial tachycardia (MAT).

TABLE **4-2**	CHARACTERISTICS OF WANDERING ATRIAL PACEMAKER (MULTIFORMED ATRIAL RHYTHM)
Rate	Usually 60-100 beats/min but may be slow; if the rate is greater than 100 beats/min, the rhythm is termed *multifocal (or chaotic) atrial tachycardia*
Rhythm	May be irregular as the pacemaker site shifts from the SA node to ectopic atrial locations and the AV junction
P waves	Size, shape, and direction may change from beat to beat; at least three different P wave configurations are required for a diagnosis of wandering atrial pacemaker or multifocal atrial tachycardia
PR interval	Variable
QRS duration	Usually less than 0.10 sec unless an intraventricular conduction delay exists

Causes and Clinical Significance

Multifocal atrial tachycardia is most commonly observed in elderly individuals and in persons with severe chronic obstructive pulmonary disease (COPD), acute myocardial infarction, hypoxia, and theophylline toxicity. Also electrolyte imbalances, such as hypokalemia and hypomagnesemia, have been reported as the etiology of this dysrhythmia.[2]

Intervention

Treatment of MAT is directed at the underlying cause. If the patient is stable but symptomatic and has normal cardiac function, interventions may include medications such as calcium channel blockers, beta-blockers, or amiodarone. Carotid sinus pressure has no effect on MAT. Treatment of the stable but symptomatic patient with impaired cardiac function may include the use of amiodarone or diltiazem.

SUPRAVENTRICULAR TACHYCARDIA (SVT)

The term **supraventricular tachycardia (SVT)** may be used in two ways. First, it describes all tachydysrhythmias that originate above the bifurcation of the bundle of His. Thus SVTs can include sinus tachycardia, atrial tachycardia, atrial flutter, atrial fibrillation, and junctional tachycardia. Second, the term refers to a dysrhythmia with a rapid ventricular rate (tachycardia) and a narrow-QRS complex, but whose specific origin (atrial or junctional) is uncertain.

The term **paroxysmal** is used to describe the sudden onset or cessation of a dysrhythmia. Correct use of the term *paroxysmal* requires observing the onset or cessation of the dysrhythmia and identification of the underlying rhythm that preceded it. An SVT that starts or ends suddenly is called **paroxysmal supraventricular tachycardia (PSVT)** (Figure 4-6). In PSVT, the QRS is narrow unless there is an intraventricular conduction delay (bundle branch block) (Table 4-3).

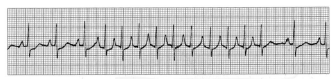

FIGURE **4-6** Paroxysmal supraventricular tachycardia (PSVT).

TABLE **4-3**	CHARACTERISTICS OF SUPRAVENTRICULAR TACHYCARDIA (SVT)
Rate	150-250 beats/min
Rhythm	Regular
P waves	Atrial P waves may be observed that differ from sinus P waves
PR interval	If P waves are seen, the PRI will usually measure 0.12-0.20 sec
QRS duration	Less than 0.10 sec unless an intraventricular conduction delay exists

Atrial Tachycardia

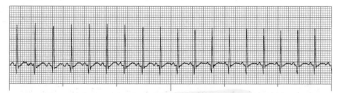

FIGURE **4-7** Atrial tachycardia.

TABLE **4-4**	CHARACTERISTICS OF ATRIAL TACHYCARDIA
Rate	150-250 beats/min
Rhythm	Regular
P waves	One positive P wave precedes each QRS complex in lead II but the P waves differ in shape from sinus P waves; with rapid rates, it is difficult to distinguish P waves from T waves
PR interval	May be shorter or longer than normal and may be difficult to measure because P waves may be hidden in T waves
QRS duration	0.10 sec or less unless an intraventricular conduction delay exists

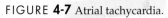

AV Nodal Reentrant Tachycardia (AVNRT)

TABLE 4-5	CHARACTERISTICS OF AV NODAL REENTRANT TACHYCARDIA (AVNRT)
Rate	150-250 beats/min; typically 170-250 beats/min
Rhythm	Ventricular rhythm is usually very regular
P waves	P waves are often hidden in the QRS complex; if the ventricles are stimulated first and then the atria, a negative (inverted) P wave will appear after the QRS in leads II, III, and aVF; when the atria are depolarized after the ventricles, the P wave typically distorts the end of the QRS complex
PR interval	P waves are not seen before the QRS complex; therefore, the PR interval is not measurable
QRS duration	Less than 0.10 sec unless an intraventricular conduction delay exists

Causes and Clinical Significance

AVNRT (Table 4-5) is common in young, healthy individuals with no structural heart disease as well as in individuals with atherosclerotic or hypertensive heart disease. AVNRT is often precipitated by a premature complex. The primary symptom during AVNRT is palpitations. Rapid ventricular rates may be associated with lightheadedness, dyspnea, weakness, nervousness, chest pain or pressure, nausea, diaphoresis, dizziness, syncope, and possible signs of shock, depending on the duration and rate of the tachycardia and the presence of structural heart disease. Recurrent episodes vary in frequency, duration, and severity from several times a day to every 2 to 3 years.

Intervention

Intervention depends on the severity of the patient's signs and symptoms. Stable but symptomatic patients are treated with oxygen therapy, IV access, and vagal maneuvers such as coughing, gagging, holding one's breath, bearing down (Valsalva maneuver), or carotid sinus pressure. When vagal maneuvers are performed, baroreceptors in the carotid arteries are stimulated to slow AV conduction, resulting in slowing of the heart rate (Box 4-2). If vagal maneuvers do not slow the rate or cause conversion of the tachycardia to a sinus rhythm, pharmacologic treatment may be necessary.

BOX 4-2   VAGAL MANEUVERS

Vagal maneuvers are methods used to stimulate baroreceptors located in the internal carotid arteries and the aortic arch. Stimulation of these receptors results in reflex stimulation of the vagus nerve and release of acetylcholine. Acetylcholine slows conduction through the AV node, resulting in slowing of the heart rate.

Examples of vagal maneuvers include:
- Coughing
- Bearing down
- Squatting
- Breath-holding
- Carotid sinus pressure
- Immersion of the face in ice water
- Stimulation of the gag reflex

Carotid pressure should be avoided in older patients. Simultaneous, bilateral carotid pressure should **never** be performed.

Signs and symptoms of hemodynamic compromise include shock, chest pain, hypotension, shortness of breath, pulmonary congestion, congestive heart failure, acute MI, and/or decreased level of consciousness. The unstable patient should be treated with oxygen therapy, IV access, consideration of medication administration, possible sedation (if awake and time permits), followed by synchronized cardioversion (Box 4-3).

Recurrent AVNRT may require treatment with a long-acting calcium channel blocker (sustained-release verapamil, long-acting diltiazem) or long-acting beta-blockers. Class Ia (procainamide

BOX 4-3   ELECTRICAL THERAPY: SYNCHRONIZED
            CARDIOVERSION

DESCRIPTION AND PURPOSE

Synchronized cardioversion reduces the potential for delivery of energy during the vulnerable period of the T wave (relative refractory period). A synchronizing circuit allows the delivery of a countershock to be "programmed." The machine searches for the highest (R wave deflection) or deepest (QS deflection) part of the QRS complex and delivers the shock a few milliseconds after this portion of the complex.

INDICATIONS (UNSTABLE PATIENT)

• Supraventricular tachycardia
• Atrial fibrillation
• Atrial flutter
• Ventricular tachycardia with a pulse

PROCEDURE

1. Administer sedation if the patient is awake and time permits.
2. Apply conductive material to the defibrillator paddles (gel) or chest wall (disposable defibrillator pads). Remove nitroglycerin paste/patches from the patient's chest if present.
3. Turn on the defibrillator.
4. Select the appropriate energy level for the clinical situation/dysrhythmia.
5. Press the synchronizer switch/button.
6. Ensure machine sensing of the QRS complex.
7. Place the defibrillator paddles (or self-adhesive defib pads) on the patient's chest. If using manual defibrillator paddles, apply firm pressure.
8. Charge the paddles and recheck the ECG rhythm.
9. LOOK (360 degrees) to be sure the area is clear. Call "Clear!"
10. Depress both discharge buttons on the paddles simultaneously to deliver the shock.
11. Reassess the ECG rhythm and patient.

and quinidine) or Class Ic (propafenone and flecainide) antidysrhythmic medications may also be used. Patients who are resistant to drug therapy or who do not wish to remain on life-long medications for AVNRT are candidates for radiofrequency catheter ablation.

AV Reentrant Tachycardia (AVRT)

The next most common type of PSVT is AV reentrant tachycardia (AVRT). **Preexcitation** is a term used to describe rhythms that originate from above the ventricles but in which the impulse travels via a pathway other than the AV node and bundle of His. Thus the supraventricular impulse excites the ventricles earlier than would be expected if the impulse traveled by way of the normal conduction system. Patients with preexcitation syndromes are prone to AVRT.

During fetal development, strands of myocardial tissue form connections between the atria and ventricles, outside the normal conduction system. These strands normally become nonfunctional shortly after birth; however, in patients with preexcitation syndrome, these connections persist as congenital malformations of working myocardial tissue. Because these connections bypass part or all of the normal conduction system, they are called **accessory pathways.** The term **bypass tract** is used when one end of an accessory pathway is attached to normal conductive tissue. This pathway may connect the right atrial and ventricular walls, the left atrial and ventricular walls, or connect the atrial and ventricular septa on either the right or the left side.

There are three major forms of preexcitation syndrome, each differentiated by its accessory pathway or bypass tract[6] (Figure 4-8):

1. In **Wolff-Parkinson-White (WPW) syndrome,** the accessory pathway is called the *Kent bundle.* It connects the atria directly to the ventricles, completely bypassing the normal conduction system (Figure 4-9 and Table 4-6).
2. In **Lown-Ganong-Levine (LGL) syndrome,** the accessory pathway is called the *James bundle.* This bundle connects the atria directly to the lower portion of the AV node, thus partially bypassing the AV node. In LGL syndrome, one end of the James bundle is attached to normal conductive tissue. This congenital pathway may be called a *bypass tract.*

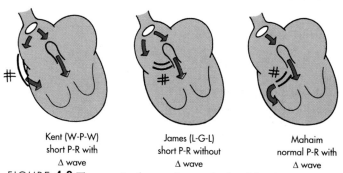

Kent (W-P-W)	James (L-G-L)	Mahaim
short P-R with	short P-R without	normal P-R with
Δ wave	Δ wave	Δ wave

FIGURE **4-8** Three major forms of preexcitation. Note location of the accessory pathways and corresponding ECG characteristics.

3. Another unnamed preexcitation syndrome involves the Mahaim fibers. These fibers do not bypass the AV node but originate below the AV node and insert into the ventricular wall, bypassing part or all of the ventricular conduction system.

Causes and Clinical Significance

Individuals with preexcitation syndrome are predisposed to tachydysrhythmias because there is a loss of the protective blocking mechanism provided by the AV node and because the accessory pathway provides a mechanism for reentry. Signs and symptoms associated with rapid ventricular rates may include palpitations, anxiety, weakness, dizziness, chest pain, shortness of breath, and shock.

PSVT and atrial fibrillation are the two most common tachydysrhythmias seen in WPW. Atrial fibrillation and atrial flutter that occur in the presence of an accessory pathway are particularly dangerous because of the extremely rapid ventricular rate than can result from conduction of the atrial impulses directly into the ventricles. The ventricular rate can be 250 to 300 beats/min and can deteriorate into ventricular fibrillation, resulting in sudden death.[7]

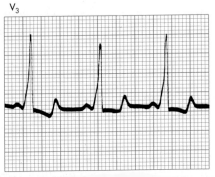

FIGURE 4-9 Typical WPW pattern showing the short PR interval, delta wave, wide QRS complex, and secondary ST and T-wave changes.

TABLE 4-6	CHARACTERISTICS OF WOLFF-PARKINSON-WHITE (WPW) SYNDROME
Rate	Usually 60-100 beats/min if the underlying rhythm is sinus in origin
Rhythm	Regular, unless associated with atrial fibrillation
P waves	Normal and positive in lead II unless WPW is associated with atrial fibrillation
PR interval	If P waves are observed, less than 0.12 sec
QRS duration	Usually greater than 0.12 sec; slurred upstroke of the QRS complex (delta wave) may be seen in one or more leads

Intervention

The stable but symptomatic patient with AVRT may be managed with oxygen therapy, IV access, attempts to slow or convert the rhythm with vagal maneuvers, and, if unsuccessful, administration of amiodarone. Medications used to slow AV conduction such as digoxin and verapamil should be **avoided** because they may accelerate the speed of conduction through the accessory pathway, resulting in a further increase in heart rate. If the patient presents with signs and symptoms of hemodynamic compromise because of the rapid ventricular rate, preparations should be made for synchronized cardioversion.

ATRIAL FLUTTER

Atrial flutter (Figure 4-10 and Table 4-7) is an ectopic atrial rhythm in which an irritable site depolarizes regularly at an extremely rapid rate. Atrial flutter has been classified into two types. Type I atrial flutter is caused by a reentrant circuit that is localized in the right atrium. Type I atrial flutter is also called *typical* or *classical atrial flutter.* Type II atrial flutter is called *atypical* or *very rapid atrial flutter.* Patients with type II atrial flutter often develop atrial fibrillation. The precise mechanism of type II atrial flutter has not been defined.

TABLE 4-7	CHARACTERISTICS OF ATRIAL FLUTTER
Rate	Atrial rate 250-450 beats/min, typically 300 beats/min; ventricular rate variable—determined by AV blockade; ventricular rate will usually not exceed 180 beats/min because of intrinsic conduction rate of AV junction
Rhythm	Atrial regular, ventricular regular or irregular depending on AV conduction/blockade
P waves	No identifiable P waves; saw-toothed "flutter" waves are present
PR interval	Not measurable
QRS duration	Usually less than 0.10 sec but may be widened if flutter waves are buried in the QRS complex or an intraventricular conduction delay exists

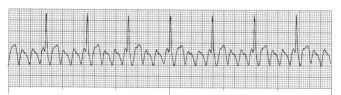

FIGURE **4-10** Atrial flutter.

Causes and Clinical Significance

Atrial flutter is usually a paroxysmal rhythm precipitated by a PAC that may last for seconds to hours and occasionally 24 hours or more. Chronic atrial flutter is unusual because the rhythm usually reverts to sinus rhythm or atrial fibrillation, either spontaneously or with treatment.[8]

The severity of signs and symptoms associated with atrial flutter vary, depending on the ventricular rate, the duration of the dysrhythmia, and the patient's cardiovascular status. The more rapid the ventricular rate, the more likely the patient is to be symptomatic with this dysrhythmia. The patient may be asymptomatic and not require treatment or may experience serious signs and symptoms and complain of palpitations or skipped beats, weakness, dizziness, or chest pressure/pain.

Intervention

When atrial flutter is present with 2:1 conduction, it may be difficult to differentiate the dysrhythmia from sinus tachycardia, atrial tachycardia, AV nodal reentrant tachycardia, AV reentrant tachycardia, or PSVT. Vagal maneuvers may help identify the rhythm by temporarily slowing AV conduction and revealing the underlying flutter waves.

In cases of atrial flutter associated with a rapid ventricular rate, treatment is first directed toward controlling the ventricular response. If cardiac function is normal, medications such as calcium channel blockers (e.g., diltiazem, verapamil) or beta-blockers (e.g., esmolol, metoprolol, propranolol) should be used. If cardiac function is impaired, medications such as digoxin, diltiazem, or amiodarone may be used.

If the patient exhibits serious signs and symptoms (shortness of breath, chest pain, hypotension, decreased level of consciousness, acute MI, congestive heart failure) because of the rapid ventricular rate, synchronized cardioversion may be performed. Atrial flutter may convert to a sinus rhythm with as little as 25 joules, although at least 50 joules is generally recommended.

ATRIAL FIBRILLATION (AFIB)

Atrial fibrillation (Afib) occurs because of multiple reentry circuits in the atria. This dysrhythmia may occur acutely (lasting less than 48 hours), paroxysmally (intermittent), or chronically (lasting at least 1 month). In atrial fibrillation, the atria are depolarized at a rate of 400 to 600 beats/min. These rapid impulses cause the muscles of the atria to quiver (fibrillate), resulting in ineffectual atrial contraction, a subsequent decrease in cardiac output, and loss of atrial kick.

Because of the quivering of the atrial muscle and because there is no uniform wave of atrial depolarization in atrial fibrillation, there is no P wave. Instead, the baseline is erratic (wavy) in appearance, corresponding with the atrial rate of 400 to 600 beats/min. These wavy deflections are called "fibrillatory" waves (Figure 4-11).

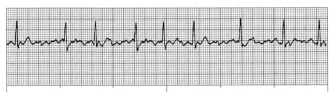

FIGURE **4-11** Atrial fibrillation.

In Afib, atrial depolarization occurs very irregularly, and the ventricular response (rhythm) is usually very irregular. The ventricular rhythm associated with atrial fibrillation is described as *irregularly irregular*. When the ventricular rate is less than 100 beats/min, atrial fibrillation is termed *controlled*. When above 100 beats/min, it is called *uncontrolled*.

Afib can occur simultaneously with complete AV block. The resulting ventricular rhythm will be slow and regular (Figure 4-12 and Table 4-8). Consider digitalis toxicity when atrial fibrillation is accompanied by a slow ventricular rate.

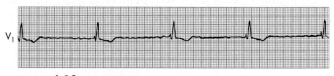

FIGURE **4-12** Atrial fibrillation with complete AV block. Ventricular rate is slow and regular because of the block.

TABLE **4-8**	CHARACTERISTICS OF ATRIAL FIBRILLATION
Rate	Atrial rate usually greater than 400-600 beats/min; ventricular rate variable
Rhythm	Ventricular rhythm usually irregularly irregular
P waves	No identifiable P waves; fibrillatory waves present; erratic, wavy baseline
PR interval	Not measurable
QRS duration	Usually less than 0.10 sec but may be widened if an intraventricular conduction delay exists

Causes and Clinical Significance

Conditions commonly associated with atrial fibrillation include rheumatic heart disease, coronary artery disease, hypertension, mitral or tricuspid valve disease, congestive heart failure, pericarditis, pulmonary embolism, cardiomyopathy, and hypoxia. Other precipitants of atrial fibrillation include drugs or intoxicants (e.g., alcohol, carbon monoxide), acute or chronic pulmonary disease, enhanced vagal tone, enhanced sympathetic tone, hypokalemia, and hyperthyroidism. Paroxysmal atrial fibrillation has been associated with excessive alcohol consumption in otherwise healthy individuals ("holiday heart syndrome").[9]

Patients experiencing Afib may develop intra-atrial emboli because the atria are not contracting, and blood stagnates in the atrial chambers. This predisposes the patient to systemic emboli, particularly stroke, if the clots dislodge spontaneously or because of conversion to a sinus rhythm. It is estimated that 15% to 20% of strokes in patients without rheumatic heart disease are the result of atrial fibrillation, and the incidence is even higher for those with rheumatic heart disease.[10]

The severity of signs and symptoms associated with atrial fibrillation vary, depending on the ventricular rate, the duration of the dysrhythmia, and the patient's cardiovascular status. The more rapid the ventricular rate, the more likely the patient is to be symptomatic with this dysrhythmia.

The patient may be asymptomatic or may experience serious signs and symptoms. Atrial fibrillation with a rapid ventricular response may produce signs and symptoms that include lightheadedness, palpitations, dyspnea, chest pressure/pain, and hypotension.

Intervention

In the stable patient with atrial fibrillation associated with a rapid ventricular rate, treatment is first directed toward controlling the ventricular response, rather than converting the dysrhythmia to a sinus rhythm. If cardiac function is normal, medications such as calcium channel blockers or beta-blockers may be used. If cardiac function is impaired, medications such as digoxin, diltiazem, or amiodarone may be used.

If the patient exhibits serious signs and symptoms (shortness of breath, chest pain, hypotension, decreased level of consciousness, acute MI, congestive heart failure) because of the rapid ventricular rate, synchronized cardioversion may be considered.

CHAPTER 5

Junctional Rhythms

The **AV node** is a group of specialized cells located in the lower portion of the right atrium, above the base of the tricuspid valve. The main function of the AV node is to delay the electrical impulse to allow the atria to contract and complete filling of the ventricles with blood before the next ventricular contraction.

After passing through the AV node, the electrical impulse enters the bundle of His. The bundle of His is located in the upper portion of the interventricular septum and connects the AV node with the two bundle branches. The bundle of His has pacemaker cells that are capable of discharging at a rhythmic rate of 40 to 60 beats/min. The AV node and the nonbranching portion of the **bundle of His** are called the **AV junction** (Figure 5-1). The bundle of His conducts the electrical impulse to the right and left bundle branches.

The AV junction may assume responsibility for pacing the heart if:

- The SA node fails to discharge (e.g., sinus arrest)
- An impulse from the SA node is generated but blocked as it exits the SA node (e.g., SA block)
- The rate of discharge of the SA node is slower than that of the AV junction (e.g., sinus bradycardia or the slower phase of a sinus arrhythmia)

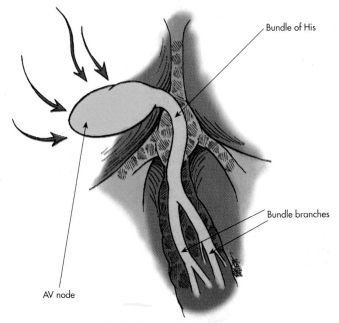

FIGURE 5-1 AV junction.

- An impulse from the SA node is generated and is conducted through the atria but is not conducted to the ventricles (e.g., AV block)

If the AV junction paces the heart, the electrical impulse must travel in a backward (retrograde) direction to activate the atria. If atrial depolarization occurs before ventricular depolarization, an inverted P wave will be seen *before* the QRS complex in leads II, III, and aVF (because the electrical impulse is traveling away from the positive electrode), and the PR interval will usually measure 0.12 sec or less. If atrial and ventricular depolarization occur simultaneously, the P wave will not be visible because it will be hidden in the QRS complex. If atrial depolarization occurs after ventricular depolarization, an inverted P wave will appear *after* the QRS complex.

PREMATURE JUNCTIONAL COMPLEXES (PJCs)

A premature junctional complex (PJC) arises from an ectopic focus within the AV junction that discharges before the next expected sinus beat (Figure 5-2 and Table 5-1). Because the impulse is conducted through the ventricles in the usual manner, the QRS complex will usually measure 0.10 sec or less. A non-compensatory (incomplete) pause often follows a PJC and represents the delay during which the SA node resets its rhythm for the next beat.

TABLE 5-1	CHARACTERISTICS OF PREMATURE JUNCTIONAL COMPLEXES (PJCs)
Rate	Usually within normal range but depends on underlying rhythm
Rhythm	Regular with premature beats
P waves	May occur before, during, or after the QRS; if visible, the P wave is inverted in leads II, III, and aVF
PR interval	If a P wave occurs before the QRS, the PR interval will usually be less than or equal to 0.12 sec; if no P wave occurs before the QRS, there will be no PR interval
QRS duration	Usually 0.10 sec or less unless an intraventricular conduction delay exists

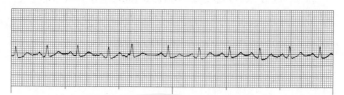

FIGURE 5-2 Lead II. Sinus tachycardia with a PJC. Rhythm strip is from a 76-year-old female complaining of shortness of breath.

Causes and Clinical Significance

PJCs are less common than either PACs or PVCs. PJCs may be caused by excessive caffeine, tobacco, or alcohol intake; valvular disease; ischemia; congestive heart failure; digitalis toxicity; increased vagal tone; acute myocardial infarction; hypoxia; electrolyte imbalance (particularly magnesium and potassium); exercise; and rheumatic heart disease.

Most individuals with PJCs are asymptomatic. However, PJCs may lead to symptoms of palpitations or the feeling of skipped beats. The sensation of skipped beats may be caused by ineffective contraction resulting from poor filling of the left ventricle during the premature beat.[8] Lightheadedness, dizziness, and other signs of decreased cardiac output may be evident if PJCs are frequent.

Intervention

PJCs do not normally require treatment. Because the rhythm is irregular, count the patient's pulse for a full minute. If PJCs occur because of ingestion of stimulants or digitalis toxicity, these substances should be withheld.

JUNCTIONAL ESCAPE BEATS/RHYTHM

A junctional escape beat originates in the AV junction and appears *late* (after the next expected sinus beat) (Figure 5-3 and Table 5-2). A junctional escape **rhythm** is several sequential junctional escape beats (Figure 5-4 and Table 5-3). Junctional escape beats and rhythms occur when the SA node fails to pace the heart or AV conduction fails. Junctional escape rhythms occur at a very regular rate of 40 to 60 beats/min.

Causes and Clinical Significance

Junctional escape beats frequently occur during episodes of sinus arrest or following pauses of nonconducted PACs.

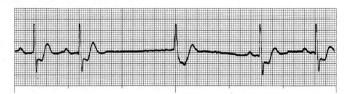

FIGURE **5-3** Sinus rhythm at 71 beats/min with a prolonged PR interval (0.24 sec), 3.36 period of sinus arrest, and a junctional escape beat.

TABLE **5-2**	CHARACTERISTICS OF JUNCTIONAL ESCAPE BEATS
Rate	Usually within normal range but depends on underlying rhythm
Rhythm	Regular with *late* beats
P waves	May occur before, during, or after the QRS; if visible, the P wave is inverted in leads II, III, and aVF
PR interval	If a P wave occurs before the QRS, the PR interval will usually be less than or equal to 0.12 sec; if no P wave occurs before the QRS, there will be no PR interval
QRS duration	Usually 0.10 sec or less unless an intraventricular conduction delay exists

Junctional escape beats may also be observed in healthy individuals during sinus bradycardia. A junctional rhythm may be seen in acute myocardial infarction (particularly inferior wall MI), rheumatic heart disease, valvular disease, disease of the SA node, hypoxia, increased parasympathetic tone, immediate post-cardiac surgery, and in patients taking digitalis, quinidine, beta-blockers, or calcium channel blockers.

The patient may be asymptomatic with a junctional escape rhythm or may experience signs and symptoms that may be associated with the slow heart rate and decreased cardiac output. Signs and symptoms may include weakness, chest pain or pressure, syncope, an altered level of consciousness, and hypotension.

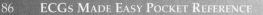

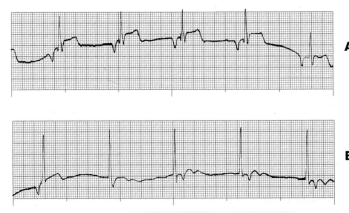

FIGURE **5-4** Junctional escape rhythm. Lead II: continuous strips. **A,** Note the retrograde P waves before the QRS complexes. **B,** Note the change in the location of the P waves. In the first beat, the retrograde P wave is observed before the QRS. In the second beat, no P wave is observed. In the remaining beats, the P wave is observed after the QRS complexes.

TABLE **5-3**	CHARACTERISTICS OF JUNCTIONAL ESCAPE RHYTHM
Rate	40-60 beats/min
Rhythm	Very regular
P waves	May occur before, during, or after the QRS; if visible, the P wave is inverted in leads II, III, and aVF
PR interval	If a P wave occurs before the QRS, the PR interval will usually be less than or equal to 0.12 sec; if no P wave occurs before the QRS, there will be no PR interval
QRS duration	Usually 0.10 sec or less unless an intraventricular conduction delay exists

Intervention

Treatment depends on the cause of the dysrhythmia and the patient's presenting signs and symptoms. If the dysrhythmia is caused by digitalis toxicity, this medication should be withheld. If the patient's signs and symptoms are related to the slow heart rate, atropine sulfate and/or transcutaneous pacing should be considered. Other medications that may be used in the treatment of symptomatic bradycardia include dopamine and epinephrine intravenous infusions.

Accelerated Junctional Rhythm

An accelerated junctional rhythm is an ectopic rhythm caused by enhanced automaticity of the bundle of His, resulting in a regular ventricular response at a rate of 60 to 100 beats/min. The ECG criteria for an accelerated junctional rhythm are the same as a junctional escape rhythm (Figure 5-5). The only difference between the two rhythms is the increase in the ventricular rate (Table 5-4).

TABLE 5-4	Characteristics of Accelerated Junctional Rhythm
Rate	61-100 beats/min
Rhythm	Very regular
P waves	May occur before, during, or after the QRS; if visible, the P wave is inverted in leads II, III, and aVF
PR interval	If a P wave occurs before the QRS, the PR interval will usually be less than or equal to 0.12 sec; if no P wave occurs before the QRS, there will be no PR interval
QRS duration	Usually 0.10 sec or less unless an intraventricular conduction delay exists

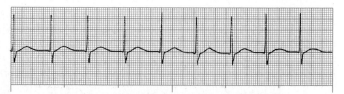

FIGURE 5-5 Accelerated junctional rhythm.

Causes and Clinical Significance

Causes of this dysrhythmia include digitalis toxicity, acute myocardial infarction, cardiac surgery, rheumatic fever, COPD, and hypokalemia. The patient may be asymptomatic with this dysrhythmia because the ventricular rate is 60 to 100 beats/min; however, the patient should be monitored closely.

Intervention

If this dysrhythmia is caused by digitalis toxicity, this medication should be withheld.

JUNCTIONAL TACHYCARDIA

TABLE 5-5	CHARACTERISTICS OF JUNCTIONAL TACHYCARDIA
Rate	101-180 beats/min
Rhythm	Very regular
P waves	May occur before, during, or after the QRS; if visible, the P wave is inverted in leads II, III, and aVF
PR interval	If a P wave occurs before the QRS, the PR interval will usually be less than or equal to 0.12 sec; if no P wave occurs before the QRS, there will be no PR interval
QRS duration	Usually 0.10 sec or less unless an intraventricular conduction delay exists

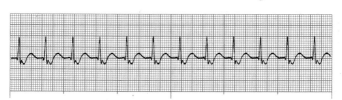

FIGURE 5-6 Junctional tachycardia.

Causes and Clinical Significance

Junctional tachycardia is an ectopic rhythm that originates in the pacemaker cells found in the bundle of His. This dysrhythmia is believed to be caused by enhanced automaticity and may occur because of myocardial ischemia or infarction, congestive heart failure, or digitalis toxicity.

With sustained ventricular rates of 150 beats/min or more, the patient may complain of a sudden feeling of a "racing heart" and severe anxiety. Because of the fast ventricular rate, the ventricles may be unable to fill completely, resulting in decreased cardiac output. Junctional tachycardia associated with acute myocardial infarction may increase myocardial ischemia and the frequency and severity of chest pain; extend the size of the infarction; cause congestive heart failure, hypotension, cardiogenic shock; and/or predispose the patient to ventricular dysrhythmias.

Intervention

Treatment depends on the severity of the patient's signs and symptoms. Signs and symptoms of hemodynamic compromise include shock, chest pain, hypotension, shortness of breath, pulmonary congestion, congestive heart failure, acute MI, and/or decreased level of consciousness.

Symptomatic patients with stable vital signs and normal cardiac function are treated with oxygen therapy, IV access, vagal maneuvers (coughing, bearing down) and, if unsuccessful, administration of adenosine. If adenosine administration is unsuccessful, amiodarone, a beta-blocker, or a calcium channel blocker may be used.

Symptomatic patients with impaired cardiac function may be treated with amiodarone.

CHAPTER 6

Ventricular Rhythms

The ventricles are the heart's least efficient pacemaker and normally generate impulses at a rate of 20 to 40 beats/min. The ventricles may assume responsibility for pacing the heart if:

- SA node fails to discharge
- Impulse from the SA node is generated but blocked as it exits the SA node
- Rate of discharge of the SA node is slower than that of the ventricles
- Irritable site in either ventricle produces an early beat or rapid rhythm

Ventricular beats and rhythms may originate from any part of the ventricles. When an ectopic site within a ventricle assumes responsibility for pacing the heart, the electrical impulse bypasses the normal intraventricular conduction pathway, and stimulation of the ventricles occurs asynchronously.

As a result, ventricular beats and rhythms are typically characterized by QRS complexes that are abnormally shaped and prolonged (greater than 0.12 sec).

Premature Ventricular Complexes (PVCs)

A **premature ventricular complex (PVC)** arises from an irritable focus within either ventricle. PVCs may be caused by enhanced automaticity or reentry. By definition, a PVC is *premature,* occurring earlier than the next expected sinus beat. The QRS of a PVC is typically equal to or greater than 0.12 sec because the PVC depolarizes the ventricles prematurely and in an abnormal manner. The T wave is usually in the opposite direction of the QRS complex (Table 6-1).

TABLE 6-1	CHARACTERISTICS OF PREMATURE VENTRICULAR COMPLEXES (PVCs)
Rate	Usually within normal range but depends on underlying rhythm
Rhythm	Essentially regular with premature beats; if the PVC is an interpolated PVC, the rhythm will be regular
P waves	Usually absent or, with retrograde conduction to the atria, may appear after the QRS (usually upright in the ST segment or T wave)
PR interval	None with the PVC because the ectopic beat originates in the ventricles
QRS duration	Greater than 0.12 sec, wide and bizarre, T wave frequently in opposite direction of the QRS complex

Types of PVCs

PVCs may occur in patterns:

- Pairs (couplets): Two sequential PVCs
- Runs or bursts: Three or more sequential PVCs, known as *ventricular tachycardia (VT)*
- Bigeminal PVCs (ventricular bigeminy): Every other beat is a PVC
- Trigeminal PVCs (ventricular trigeminy): Every third beat is a PVC

- Quadrigeminal PVCs (ventricular quadrigeminy): Every fourth beat is a PVC

Uniform and Multiformed PVCs

Premature ventricular beats that look the same in the same lead and originate from the same anatomic site (focus) are called **uniform** PVCs (Figure 6-1). PVCs that appear different from one another in the same lead are called **multiform** PVCs (Figure 6-2). Multiform PVCs often, but do not always, arise from different anatomic sites. The terms *unifocal* and *multifocal* are sometimes used to describe PVCs that are similar or different in appearance. Uniform PVCs are unifocal, but multiform PVCs are not necessarily multifocal.[9]

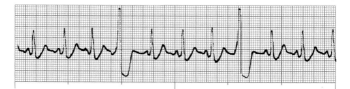

FIGURE **6-1** Sinus tachycardia with frequent uniform PVCs.

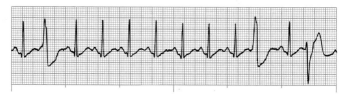

FIGURE **6-2** Sinus tachycardia with multiform PVCs.

Interpolated PVCs

A PVC may occur without interfering with the normal cardiac cycle. An **interpolated PVC** (Figure 6-3) does not have a full compensatory pause—it is "squeezed" between two regular complexes and does not disturb the underlying rhythm. The PR interval of the cardiac cycle following the PVC may be longer than normal.

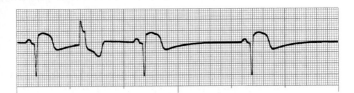

FIGURE **6-3** Sinus bradycardia with an interpolated PVC and ST-segment elevation.

R-on-T PVCs

R-on-T PVCs occur when the R wave of a PVC falls on the T wave of the preceding beat (Figure 6-4). Because the T wave is vulnerable (relative refractory period) to any electrical stimulation, it is possible that a PVC occurring during this period of the cardiac cycle will precipitate VT or VF; however, VT and VF most commonly occur without a preceding R-on-T PVC, and most R-on-T PVCs do not precipitate a sustained ventricular tachydysrhythmia.[9]

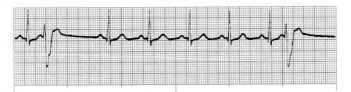

FIGURE **6-4** Sinus rhythm with two R-on-T PVCs.

Paired PVCs (Couplets)

A pair of PVCs occurring in immediate succession is called **couplet** or **paired** PVCs (Figure 6-5). The appearance of couplets indicates the ventricular ectopic site is extremely irritable. Three or more PVCs occurring in immediate succession at a rate of more than 100 beats/min is considered a "salvo," "run," or "burst" of ventricular tachycardia.

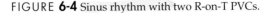

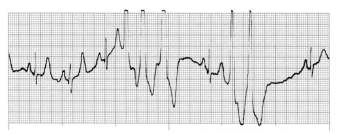

FIGURE **6-5** Sinus rhythm with a run of VT and one episode of couplets.

Causes and Clinical Significance

PVCs can occur in healthy persons with apparently normal hearts and for no apparent cause. PVCs may occur because of hypoxia, stress, an increase in catecholamines, stimulants (alcohol, caffeine, tobacco), acid-base imbalance, electrolyte imbalance, digitalis toxicity, medications (epinephrine, dopamine, phenothiazines, isoproterenol), ischemia, myocardial infarction, or congestive heart failure.

PVCs may or may not produce palpable pulses. Patients experiencing PVCs may be asymptomatic or complain of palpitations, a "racing heart," skipped beats, or chest or neck discomfort.

Intervention

Treatment of PVCs depends on the cause, patient's signs and symptoms, and on the clinical situation. Most patients experiencing PVCs do not require treatment with antidysrhythmic medications. Treatment of PVCs seen in the setting of acute MI should be directed at ensuring adequate oxygenation, relief of pain, and rapid identification and correction of hypoxia, heart failure, and electrolyte or acid-base abnormalities.

Ventricular Escape Beats/Rhythm

A **ventricular escape beat** is a ventricular ectopic beat that occurs after a pause in which the supraventricular pacemakers failed to initiate an impulse. Ventricular escape beats are wide, the QRS measuring 0.12 sec or greater, and occur *late* in the cardiac cycle, appearing after the next expected sinus beat (Table 6-2). The ventricular escape beat (Figure 6-6) is a *protective* mechanism, protecting the heart from more extreme slowing or even asystole. A ventricular escape or **idioventricular rhythm (IVR)** exists when three or more sequential ventricular escape beats occur at a rate of 20 to 40 beats/min (Figure 6-7 and Table 6-3).

Causes and Clinical Significance

IVR may occur when the SA node and the AV junction fail to initiate an electrical impulse, when the rate of discharge of the SA node or AV junction becomes less than the inherent ventricular rate, or when impulses generated by a supraventricular site are blocked. IVR may also occur because of myocardial infarction, digitalis toxicity, or metabolic imbalances.

Because the ventricular rate associated with this rhythm is slow (20 to 40 beats/min) with loss of atrial kick, the patient may

TABLE 6-2	CHARACTERISTICS OF VENTRICULAR ESCAPE BEATS
Rate	Usually within normal range but depends on underlying rhythm
Rhythm	Essentially regular with late beats; the ventricular escape beat occurs after the next expected sinus beat
P waves	Usually absent or, with retrograde conduction to the atria, may appear after the QRS (usually upright in the ST segment or T wave)
PR interval	None with the ventricular escape beat because the ectopic beat originates in the ventricles
QRS duration	Greater than 0.12 sec, wide and bizarre, T wave frequently in opposite direction of the QRS complex

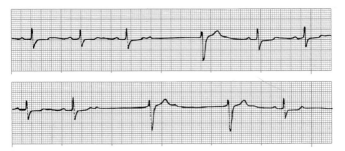

FIGURE **6-6** Ventricular escape beats following nonconducted premature atrial complexes.

TABLE **6-3**	CHARACTERISTICS OF VENTRICULAR ESCAPE (IDIOVENTRICULAR) RHYTHM
Rate	20-40 beats/min
Rhythm	Essentially regular
P waves	Usually absent or, with retrograde conduction to the atria, may appear after the QRS (usually upright in the ST segment or T wave)
PR interval	None
QRS duration	Greater than 0.12 sec, T wave frequently in opposite direction of the QRS complex

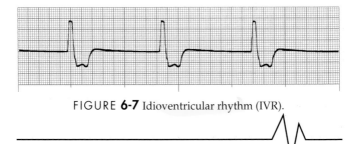

FIGURE **6-7** Idioventricular rhythm (IVR).

experience severe hypotension, weakness, disorientation, light-headedness, or loss of consciousness because of decreased cardiac output.

Intervention

Lidocaine should be *avoided* in the management of this rhythm because lidocaine may abolish ventricular activity, possibly causing asystole in a patient with an idioventricular rhythm. If the patient is symptomatic because of the slow rate and/or loss of atrial kick, atropine may be ordered in an attempt to block the vagus nerve and stimulate the SA node to overdrive the ventricular rhythm, or transcutaneous pacing may be attempted. If the patient is pulseless despite the appearance of organized electrical activity on the cardiac monitor (a clinical situation termed *pulseless electrical activity*), management should include CPR, oxygen administration and endotracheal intubation, IV access, and an aggressive search for the underlying cause of the situation.

Accelerated Idioventricular Rhythm (AIVR)

An **accelerated idioventricular rhythm (AIVR)** exists when three or more sequential ventricular escape beats occur at a rate of 41 to 100 beats/min (Figure 6-8). P waves are usually absent but, with retrograde conduction to the atria, may appear after

TABLE 6-4	Characteristics of Accelerated Idioventricular Rhythm (AIVR)
Rate	41-100 beats/min
Rhythm	Essentially regular
P waves	Usually absent or, with retrograde conduction to the atria, may appear after the QRS (usually upright in the ST segment or T wave)
PR interval	None
QRS duration	Greater than 0.12 sec, T wave frequently in opposite direction of the QRS complex

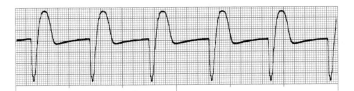

FIGURE **6-8** Accelerated idioventricular rhythm (AIVR).

the QRS (usually upright in the ST segment or T wave). The ventricular rhythm is essentially regular with a QRS that is greater than 0.12 sec in duration. The T wave is frequently in an opposite direction of the QRS complex (Table 6-4).

Causes and Clinical Significance

AIVR is usually considered a benign escape rhythm that appears when the sinus rate slows and disappears when the sinus rate speeds up. AIVR is often seen during the first 12 hours of a myocardial infarction and is particularly common after successful reperfusion therapy. AIVR is seen in both anterior and inferior MI and in 90% of patients during the first 24 hours after reperfusion.[2] AIVR has been reported in 10% to 40% of patients with acute MI,[5] in patients with digitalis toxicity, subarachnoid hemorrhage, and in patients with rheumatic and hypertensive heart disease.

Intervention

If the patient is asymptomatic, no treatment is necessary. If the patient is symptomatic because of the loss of atrial kick, atropine may be ordered in an attempt to block the vagus nerve and stimulate the SA node to overdrive the ventricular rhythm, or transcutaneous pacing may be attempted. Medications to suppress the ventricular rhythm should be avoided because this rhythm is protective and often transient, spontaneously resolving on its own.

Ventricular Tachycardia (VT)

Ventricular tachycardia (VT) (Figure 6-9) exists when three or more PVCs occur in immediate succession at a rate greater than 100 beats/min. VT may occur as a short run lasting less than 30 seconds (nonsustained) but more commonly persists for more than 30 seconds (sustained). VT may occur with or without pulses, and the patient may be stable or unstable with this rhythm.

Ventricular tachycardia, like PVCs, may originate from an ectopic focus in either ventricle. In VT, the QRS complex is wide and bizarre. P waves, if visible, bear no relationship to the QRS complex. The ventricular rhythm is usually regular but may be slightly irregular. When the QRS complexes of VT are of the same shape and amplitude, the rhythm is termed **monomorphic VT** (Table 6-5). When the QRS complexes of VT vary in shape and amplitude, the rhythm is termed **polymorphic VT**.

TABLE 6-5	CHARACTERISTICS OF MONOMORPHIC VENTRICULAR TACHYCARDIA
Rate	101-250 beats/min
Rhythm	Essentially regular
P waves	May be present or absent; if present, they have no set relationship to the QRS complexes, appearing between the QRSs at a rate different from that of the VT
PR interval	None
QRS duration	Greater than 0.12 sec; often difficult to differentiate between the QRS and T wave

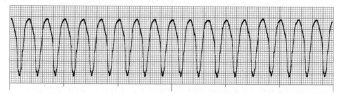

FIGURE **6-9** Monomorphic ventricular tachycardia (VT).

Causes and Clinical Significance

Sustained monomorphic VT is often associated with underlying heart disease, particularly myocardial ischemia, and rarely occurs in patients without underlying structural heart disease. The most common cause of sustained monomorphic VT in American adults is coronary artery disease with prior myocardial infarction.[9] Other causes of VT include cardiomyopathy, cyclic antidepressant overdose, digitalis toxicity, valvular heart disease, mitral valve prolapse, trauma (e.g., myocardial contusion, invasive cardiac procedures), acid-base imbalance, electrolyte imbalance (e.g., hypokalemia, hyperkalemia, hypomagnesemia), and increased production of catecholamines (e.g., fright, cocaine abuse).[2]

Signs and symptoms of hemodynamic compromise related to the tachycardia may include shock, chest pain, hypotension, shortness of breath, pulmonary congestion, congestive heart failure, acute myocardial infarction, and/or a decreased level of consciousness.

Intervention

Treatment is based on the patient's presentation. *Stable* but symptomatic patients are treated with oxygen therapy, IV access, and administration of ventricular antidysrhythmics to suppress the rhythm.

Unstable patients (usually a sustained heart rate of 150 beats/min or more) whose signs and symptoms are a result of the rapid heart rate are treated with administration of oxygen, IV access, consideration of the use of medications, sedation (if awake and time permits) followed by electrical therapy. CPR should be initiated for the pulseless patient in VT until a defibrillator is available.

POLYMORPHIC VENTRICULAR TACHYCARDIA

Polymorphic ventricular tachycardia (VT) refers to a rapid ventricular dysrhythmia with beat-to-beat changes in the shape and amplitude of the QRS complexes. Polymorphic VT that occurs in the presence of a long QT interval is called *torsades de pointes*.

Torsades de Pointes (TdP)

Torsades de pointes (TdP) is a dysrhythmia intermediary between ventricular tachycardia and ventricular fibrillation[2] and is a type of polymorphic VT associated with a prolonged QT interval. Torsades de pointes is French for "twisting of the points," which describes the QRS that changes in shape, amplitude, and width and appears to "twist" around the isoelectric line, resembling a spindle (Figure 6-10 and Table 6-6).

TABLE 6-6	CHARACTERISTICS OF TORSADES DE POINTES (TDP)
Rate	150-300 beats/min, typically 200-250 beats/min
Rhythm	May be regular or irregular
P waves	None
PR interval	None
QRS duration	Greater than 0.12 sec; gradual alteration in amplitude and direction of the QRS complexes

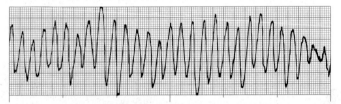

FIGURE 6-10 Torsades de pointes (TdP).

Causes and Clinical Significance
TdP may be precipitated by slow heart rates and is associated with medications or electrolyte disturbances that prolong the QT interval. Symptoms associated with TdP are usually related

to the decreased cardiac output that occurs because of the fast ventricular rate. Patients may complain of palpitations, light-headedness, or may experience a syncopal episode or seizures. TdP may be initiated by a PVC and may occasionally terminate spontaneously and recur after several seconds or minutes or may deteriorate to VF.

Intervention

Obtaining a 12-lead ECG may be helpful in identifying TdP because the rhythm may appear to be monomorphic VT in one lead but present the pattern typical of TdP in another.[2] Treatment of TdP includes discontinuation of type Ia antidysrhythmics (if drug induced), correction of electrolyte abnormalities, and any one of the following interventions: overdrive pacing, magnesium, isoproterenol, lidocaine, or phenytoin. Defibrillation may be necessary for termination of sustained episodes of TdP.

VENTRICULAR FIBRILLATION (VF)

Ventricular fibrillation (VF) is a chaotic rhythm that originates in the ventricles. In VF, there is no organized depolarization of the ventricles. The ventricular myocardium quivers and, as a result, there is no effective myocardial contraction and no pulse. The resulting rhythm is irregularly irregular with chaotic deflections that vary in shape and amplitude. No normal-looking waveforms are visible (Figures 6-11 and 6-12 and Table 6-7).

TABLE 6-7	CHARACTERISTICS OF VENTRICULAR FIBRILLATION (VF)
Rate	Cannot be determined because there are no discernible waves or complexes to measure
Rhythm	Rapid and chaotic with no pattern or regularity
P waves	Not discernible
PR interval	Not discernible
QRS duration	Not discernible

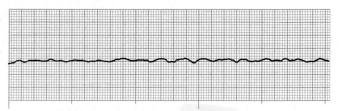

FIGURE **6-11** Fine VF.

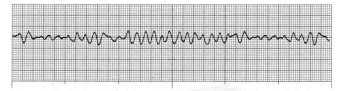

FIGURE **6-12** Coarse VF.

Causes and Clinical Significance

The patient in VF is unresponsive, apneic, and pulseless. Extrinsic factors that enhance the vulnerability of the myocardium to fibrillate include increased sympathetic nervous system activity, vagal stimulation, metabolic abnormalities (e.g., hypokalemia, hypomagnesemia), antidysrhythmics and other medications (e.g., psychotropics, digitalis, sympathomimetics), and environmental factors (e.g., electrocution). Intrinsic factors include hypertrophy, ischemia, myocardial failure, enhanced AV conduction (e.g., bypass tracts, "fast" AV node), abnormal repolarization, and bradycardia.[11]

Intervention

CPR should be initiated for the patient in VF until a defibrillator is available. On arrival of the defibrillator, unsynchronized shocks should be delivered (Box 6-1), an endotracheal tube should be placed, IV access established, and medications administered per current resuscitation guidelines.

BOX 6-1   ELECTRICAL THERAPY: DEFIBRILLATION (UNSYNCHRONIZED COUNTERSHOCK)

DESCRIPTION AND PURPOSE

The purpose of defibrillation is to produce momentary asystole. The shock attempts to completely depolarize the myocardium and provide an opportunity for the natural pacemaker centers of the heart to resume normal activity. Defibrillation is a random delivery of energy—the discharge of energy is not related to the cardiac cycle.

INDICATIONS

- Pulseless VT
- Ventricular fibrillation
- Sustained torsades de pointes
- Undue delay in delivery of synchronized cardioversion

PROCEDURE

1. Apply conductive material to the defibrillator paddles (gel) or chest wall (disposable defibrillator pads). Remove nitroglycerin paste/patches from the patient's chest if present.
2. Turn on the defibrillator.
3. Select the appropriate energy level for the clinical situation/dysrhythmia.
4. Place the defibrillator paddles (or self-adhesive defib pads) on the patient's chest. If using manual defibrillator paddles, apply firm pressure.
5. Charge the paddles and recheck the ECG rhythm.
6. LOOK (360 degrees) to be sure the area is clear. Call "Clear"!
7. Depress both discharge buttons simultaneously to deliver the shock.
8. Reassess the ECG rhythm.

ASYSTOLE (CARDIAC STANDSTILL)

TABLE 6-8	CHARACTERISTICS OF ASYSTOLE
Rate	Ventricular rate usually not discernible but atrial activity may be observed ("P-wave" asystole)
Rhythm	Ventricular not discernible, atrial may be discernible
P waves	Usually not discernible
PR interval	Not measurable
QRS duration	Absent

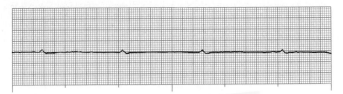

FIGURE **6-13** "P-wave" asytole.

Causes and Clinical Significance

Asystole (Figure 6-13 and Table 6-8) may occur because of extensive myocardial damage (possibly from ischemia or infarction),
hypoxia, hypokalemia, hyperkalemia, hypothermia, acidosis,
drug overdose, ventricular aneurysm, acute respiratory failure, or
traumatic cardiac arrest. Ventricular asystole may occur temporarily following termination of a tachydysrhythmia by medication
administration, defibrillation, or synchronized cardioversion.

Intervention

Treatment of asystole includes confirmation of the absence of a
pulse, immediate CPR, confirmation of the rhythm in two leads,
endotracheal intubation, IV access, consideration of the possible
causes of the rhythm, consideration of early initiation of transcutaneous pacing, and medication therapy.

PULSELESS ELECTRICAL ACTIVITY (PEA)

Pulseless electrical activity (PEA) is a clinical situation, not a
specific dysrhythmia. PEA exists when organized electrical
activity (other than VT) is observed on the cardiac monitor, but
mechanical contraction of the myocardial fibers does not occur.
Therefore, despite the presence of an organized rhythm on the
cardiac monitor, the patient is pulseless (Figure 6-14).

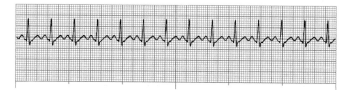

FIGURE **6-14** Rhythm shown is a sinus tachycardia; however, if no pulse is associated with the rhythm, the clinical situation is termed *pulseless electrical activity (PEA).*

BOX **6-2**   PATCH-4-MD

Possible causes of PEA:
Pulmonary embolism
Acidosis
Tension pneumothorax
Cardiac tamponade
Hypovolemia (most common cause)
Hypoxia
Heat/cold (hypo-/hyperthermia)
Hypo-/hyperkalemia (and other electrolytes)
Myocardial infarction
Drug overdose/accidents (cyclic antidepressants, calcium channel blockers, beta-blockers, digoxin)

Causes and Clinical Significance

Many conditions may cause PEA. The acronym PATCH-4-MD can be used as an aid in memorizing many of the possible causes of PEA (Box 6-2). PEA has a poor prognosis unless the underlying cause can be rapidly identified and appropriately managed.

Intervention

Treatment of PEA includes CPR, endotracheal intubation, IV access, an aggressive search for possible causes of the situation, and medications per current resuscitation guidelines.

CHAPTER 7

Atrioventricular (AV) Blocks

The **AV junction** is an area of specialized conduction tissue that provides the electrical links between the atrium and ventricle. If a delay or interruption in impulse conduction occurs within the AV node, bundle of His, or His-Purkinje system, the resulting dysrhythmia is called an *atrioventricular (AV) block.* AV blocks have been traditionally classified in two ways—according to the degree of block and/or according to the site of block (Table 7-1).

FIRST-DEGREE AV BLOCK

Causes and Clinical Significance

First-degree AV block may be a normal finding in individuals with no history of cardiac disease, especially in athletes (Figure 7-1 and Table 7-2). First-degree AV block may also occur because of ischemia or injury to the AV node or junction, medication therapy (e.g., quinidine, procainamide, beta-blockers, calcium channel blockers, digitalis, and amiodarone), rheumatic heart disease, hyperkalemia, acute myocardial infarction (often inferior wall MI), or increased vagal tone.

TABLE 7-1	CLASSIFICATION OF AV BLOCKS		
Degree of block	Incomplete blocks		First-degree AV block
			Second-degree AV block, type I
			Second-degree AV block, type II
			Second-degree AV block, 2:1 conduction
	Complete block		Complete (third-degree) AV block
Site of block	AV node		First-degree AV block
			Second-degree AV block, type I
			Complete (third-degree) AV block
	Infranodal (subnodal)	Bundle of His	Second-degree AV block, type II (uncommon)
			Complete (third-degree) AV block
		Bundle branches	Second-degree AV block, type II (more common)
			Complete (third-degree) AV block

TABLE 7-2	CHARACTERISTICS OF FIRST-DEGREE AV BLOCK
Rate	Usually within normal range but depends on underlying rhythm
Rhythm	Regular
P waves	Normal in size and shape, one positive (upright) P wave before each QRS in leads II, III, and aVF
PR interval	Prolonged (greater than 0.20 sec) but constant
QRS duration	Usually 0.10 sec or less unless an intraventricular conduction delay exists

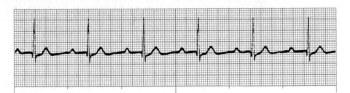

FIGURE **7-1** Sinus rhythm at 60 beats/min with a first-degree AV block.

Intervention

The patient with a first-degree AV block is often asymptomatic; however, marked first-degree AV block can lead to symptoms even in the absence of higher degrees of AV block.[12] First-degree AV block that occurs with acute myocardial infarction should be monitored closely.

SECOND-DEGREE AV BLOCKS

When some, but not all, atrial impulses are blocked from reaching the ventricles, second-degree AV block results. Because the SA node is generating impulses in a normal manner, each P wave will occur at a regular interval across the rhythm strip (all P waves will plot through on time), although not every P wave will be followed by a QRS complex. This suggests that the atria are being depolarized normally, but not every impulse is being conducted to the ventricles. As a result, more P waves than QRS complexes are visible on the ECG rhythm strip.

Second-Degree AV Block, Type I (Wenckebach, Mobitz Type I)

Causes and Clinical Significance
Second-degree AV block type I (Table 7-3 and Figure 7-2) is caused by conduction delay within the AV node and is most commonly associated with AV nodal ischemia secondary to occlusion of the

TABLE **7-3**	**CHARACTERISTICS OF SECOND-DEGREE AV BLOCK, TYPE I**
Rate	Atrial rate is greater than the ventricular rate
Rhythm	Atrial regular (P waves plot through); ventricular irregular
P waves	Normal in size and shape; some P waves are not followed by a QRS complex (more Ps than QRSs)
PR interval	Lengthens with each cycle (although lengthening may be very slight) until a P wave appears without a QRS complex; the PRI *after* the nonconducted beat is shorter than the interval preceding the nonconducted beat
QRS duration	Usually 0.10 sec or less but is periodically dropped

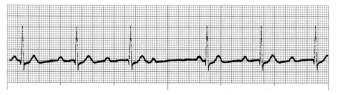

FIGURE **7-2** Second-degree AV block, type I.

right coronary artery.[8] Second-degree AV block type I may also occur because of increased parasympathetic tone or the effects of medication (e.g., digitalis, beta-blockers, verapamil). When associated with an acute inferior wall myocardial infarction, this dysrhythmia is usually transient, resolving within 48 to 72 hours as the effects of parasympathetic stimulation disappear.

Intervention
The patient with this dysrhythmia is usually asymptomatic because the ventricular rate often remains nearly normal, and

cardiac output is not significantly affected. If the patient is symptomatic and the dysrhythmia is a result of medications, these substances should be withheld. If the heart rate is slow and serious signs and symptoms (low blood pressure, shortness of breath, congestive heart failure, chest pain, pulmonary congestion, decreased level of consciousness) occur because of the slow rate, atropine and/or temporary pacing should be considered. When this dysrhythmia occurs in conjunction with acute myocardial infarction, the patient should be observed for increasing AV block.

Second-Degree AV Block, Type II (Mobitz Type II)

Causes and Clinical Significance
The bundle branches receive their primary blood supply from the left coronary artery. Thus disease of the left coronary artery or an anterior myocardial infarction is usually associated with blocks that occur within the bundle branches. Second-degree AV block type II (Table 7-4 and Figure 7-3) may also occur because of acute myocarditis or other types of organic heart disease. The patient's response to this dysrhythmia is usually related to the ventricular rate. If the ventricular rate is within normal limits, the patient may be asymptomatic. More commonly, the ventricular rate is significantly slowed and serious signs and symptoms result (low blood pressure, shortness of breath, congestive heart failure, pulmonary congestion, decreased level of consciousness) because of the slow rate and decreased cardiac output.

Intervention
Second-degree AV block type II may rapidly progress to complete AV block without warning. If the patient is symptomatic, transcutaneous pacing should be instituted until transvenous pacemaker insertion can be accomplished.

TABLE 7-4	CHARACTERISTICS OF SECOND-DEGREE AV BLOCK, TYPE II
Rate	Atrial rate is greater than the ventricular rate; ventricular rate is often slow
Rhythm	Atrial regular (P waves plot through); ventricular irregular
P waves	Normal in size and shape; some P waves are not followed by a QRS complex (more Ps than QRSs)
PR interval	Within normal limits or slightly prolonged but constant for the conducted beats; there may be some shortening of the PR interval that follows a nonconducted P wave
QRS duration	Usually 0.10 sec or greater, periodically absent after P waves

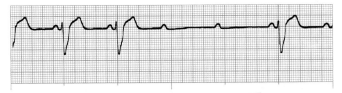

FIGURE **7-3** Second-degree AV block, type II.

Second-Degree AV Block, 2:1 Conduction (2:1 AV Block)

When two conducted P waves occur *consecutively,* the PR intervals of the consecutive beats should be compared to identify either type I or type II second-degree AV block. If two P waves occur for every one QRS complex (2:1 conduction), the decision as to what to term the rhythm is based on the width of the QRS complex.

A 2:1 AV conduction pattern associated with a narrow QRS complex (0.10 sec or less) usually represents a form of second-degree AV block, type I (Figure 7-4). A 2:1 AV conduction pattern associated with wide QRS complexes (greater than 0.10 sec) is usually associated with a delay in conduction below the bundle of His—thus it is usually a type II block (Figure 7-5 and Table 7-5).

TABLE 7-5	CHARACTERISTICS OF SECOND-DEGREE AV BLOCK, 2:1 CONDUCTION
Rate	Atrial rate is twice the ventricular rate
Rhythm	Atrial regular (P waves plot through); ventricular regular
P waves	Normal in size and shape; every other P wave is followed by a QRS complex (more Ps than QRSs)
PR interval	Constant
QRS duration	Within normal limits if the block occurs above the bundle of His (probably type I); wide if the block occurs below the bundle of His (probably type II); absent after every other P wave

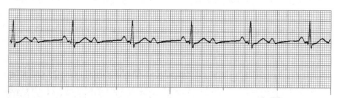

FIGURE 7-4 Second-degree AV block, 2:1 conduction, probably type I.

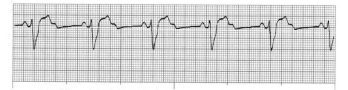

FIGURE 7-5 Second-degree AV block, 2:1 conduction, probably type II.

Causes and Clinical Significance

The causes and clinical significance of second-degree AV block with 2:1 conduction are those of type I or type II block previously described. Clinically, conduction usually improves in response to exercise or administration of atropine or catecholamines in type I AV block. In type II AV block, conduction typically worsens with exercise or administration of atropine or catecholamines.

COMPLETE AV BLOCK

First- and second-degree AV blocks are types of *incomplete blocks* because the AV junction conducts at least some impulses to the ventricles.[9] With **complete AV block,** the atria and ventricles beat independently of each other. Impulses generated by the sinoatrial node are blocked before reaching the ventricles. The block may occur at the AV node, bundle of His, or bundle branches. A secondary pacemaker (either junctional or ventricular) stimulates the ventricles; therefore, the QRS may be narrow or wide, depending on the location of the escape pacemaker and the condition of the intraventricular conduction system (Table 7-6).

TABLE 7-6	CHARACTERISTICS OF COMPLETE AV BLOCK
Rate	Atrial rate is greater than the ventricular rate; the ventricular rate is determined by the origin of the escape rhythm
Rhythm	Atrial regular (P waves plot through); ventricular regular; there is no relationship between the atrial and ventricular rhythms
P waves	Normal in size and shape
PR interval	None—the atria and ventricles beat independently of each other; thus there is no true PR interval
QRS duration	Narrow or wide, depending on the location of the escape pacemaker and the condition of the intraventricular conduction system; narrow indicates junctional pacemaker; wide indicates ventricular pacemaker

Causes and Clinical Significance

Complete AV block has an incidence of 5.8% in the early period of acute MI and is nearly twice as common with inferior/posterior infarctions compared with anterior infarction.[8] When associated with an inferior MI, complete AV block often resolves on its own within a week. Complete AV block associated with an anterior MI may develop suddenly and without warning, usually 12 to 24 hours after the onset of acute ischemia.

Generally, complete AV block with narrow QRS complexes (junctional escape pacemaker with a ventricular rate of more than 40 beats/min) (Figure 7-6) is a more stable rhythm that a complete AV block with wide QRS complexes (ventricular pacemaker with a ventricular rate that is usually less than 40 beats/min) (Figure 7-7) because the ventricular escape pacemaker is usually slower and less consistent.[9]

Intervention

The patient's signs and symptoms will depend on the origin of the escape pacemaker (junctional vs. ventricular) and the patient's response to a slower ventricular rate.

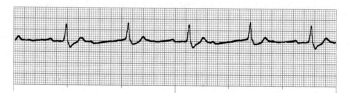

FIGURE **7-6** Complete AV block with a junctional escape pacemaker (QRS 0.08 to 0.10 sec).

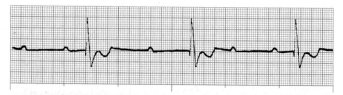

FIGURE **7-7** Complete AV block with a ventricular escape pacemaker (QRS 0.12 to 0.14 sec).

CHAPTER 8

Pacemaker Rhythms

PACEMAKER MODES

Fixed-Rate (Asynchronous) Pacemakers

A **fixed-rate pacemaker** continuously discharges at a preset rate (usually 70 to 80/min) regardless of the patient's heart rate. An advantage of the fixed-rate pacemaker is its simple circuitry, reducing the risk of pacemaker failure. This type of pacemaker does not sense the patient's own cardiac rhythm. This may result in competition between the patient's cardiac rhythm and that of the pacemaker. Ventricular tachycardia or ventricular fibrillation may be induced if the pacemaker were to fire during the T wave (vulnerable period) of a preceding patient beat. Fixed-rate pacemakers are not often used today.

Demand (Synchronous, Noncompetitive) Pacemakers

A **demand pacemaker** discharges only when the patient's heart rate drops below the pacemaker's preset (base) rate. For example, if the demand pacemaker's pulse generator were preset at a rate of 70 impulses/min, it would sense the patient's heart rate and allow electrical impulses to flow from the pacemaker through the pacing lead to stimulate the heart only when the rate fell below

70 beats/min. Demand pacemakers can be programmable or nonprogrammable. The voltage level and impulse rate are preset at the time of manufacture in nonprogrammable pacemakers.

Pacemaker Identification Codes

The Intersociety Commission on Heart Disease (ICHD), now referred to as North American British Generic (NBG), developed an international identification code in 1974 to assist in identifying a pacemaker's preprogrammed pacing, sensing, and response functions. This coding system traditionally consisted of three letters. In 1980, the system was modified to add two additional functions (letters) (Table 8-1).

The first three letters are used for antibradycardia functions. The *first letter* of the code identifies the heart chamber (or chambers) paced (stimulated). The options available include:

O, none
A, atrium
V, ventricle
D, dual (both atrium and ventricle)

A pacemaker used to pace only a single chamber is represented by either *A* (atrial) or *V* (ventricular). A pacemaker capable of pacing in both chambers is represented by *D* (dual).

The *second letter* identifies the chamber of the heart where patient-initiated (intrinsic) electrical activity is sensed by the pacemaker. The letter designations for the second letter are the same as the designations for the first.

The *third letter* indicates how the pacemaker will respond when it senses patient-initiated electrical activity:

O, no sensing
T, pacemaker stimulus is *triggered* in response to a sensed event

TABLE 8-1	PACEMAKER CODES			
Chamber paced (first letter)	Chamber sensed (second letter)	Response to sensing (third letter)	Programmable functions (fourth letter)	Antitachycardia functions (fifth letter)
O = None A = Atrium V = Ventricle D = Dual chamber (atrium and ventricle)	O = None (fixed-rate pacemaker) A = Atrium V = Ventricle D = Dual chamber (atrium and ventricle)	O = None (fixed-rate pacemaker) T = Triggers pacing I = Inhibits pacing D = Dual (triggers and inhibits pacing)	O = None P = Simple programmability (rate and/or output) M = Multi-programmable C = Communication R = Rate responsive	O = None P = Pacing (anti-tachycardia) S = Shock D = Dual (pacing and shock)

I, sensing of intrinsic impulses *inhibits* the pacemaker from producing a stimulus

D, dual (a combination of triggered pacing and inhibition)

The *fourth letter* is most often used in permanent pacing and identifies the availability of rate responsiveness and the number of reprogrammable functions available:

O, the pacemaker is not programmable or rate responsive (most commonly found on devices manufactured before the mid-1970s)

P, simple programmability where the pacemaker is limited to one or two programmable parameters (e.g., such as rate or output)

M, multiprogrammability (i.e., more than two variables can be altered)

C, capability of transmitting and/or receiving data for informational or programming purposes

R, rate responsiveness, denoting the pacemaker's ability to automatically adjust its rate to meet the body's needs caused by increased physical activity

The *fifth letter* indicates the presence of one or more active antitachycardia functions and indicates how the pacemaker will respond to tachydysrhythmias:

O, the device has no antitachycardia functions

P, the device is capable of antitachycardia pacing

S, the device is capable of delivering synchronized and unsynchronized countershocks

D, the device is capable of antitachycardia pacing, synchronized and unsynchronized countershocks

SINGLE-CHAMBER PACEMAKERS

A pacemaker that paces a single heart chamber (either the atrium or ventricle) has one lead placed in the heart. Atrial pacing is achieved by placing the pacing electrode in the right atrium.

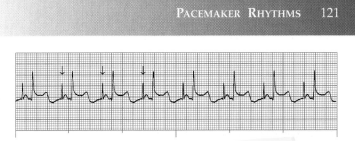

FIGURE **8-1** Atrial pacing. (*Arrows,* pacer spikes.)

Stimulation of the atria produces a pacemaker spike on the ECG followed by a P wave (Figure 8-1). Atrial pacing may be used when the SA node is diseased or damaged, but conduction through the AV junction and ventricles is normal. This type of pacemaker is ineffective if an AV block develops because it cannot pace the ventricles.

Ventricular pacing is accomplished by placing the pacing electrode in the right ventricle. Stimulation of the ventricles produces a pacemaker spike on the ECG followed by a wide QRS, resembling a ventricular ectopic bead (Figure 8-2). The QRS complex is wide because a paced impulse does not follow the normal conduction pathways in the heart.

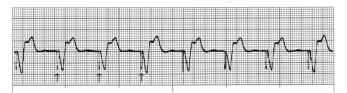

FIGURE **8-2** Ventricular pacing. (*Arrows,* pacer spikes.)

The **ventricular demand (VVI) pacemaker** is a common type of pacemaker. With this device, the pacemaker electrode is placed in the right ventricle *(V)*; the ventricle is sensed *(V)* and the pacemaker is inhibited *(I)* when spontaneous ventricular depolarization occurs within a preset interval. When spontaneous ventricular depolarization does not occur within this preset interval, the pacemaker fires and stimulates ventricular depolarization at a preset rate.

DUAL-CHAMBER PACEMAKERS

A pacemaker that paces both the atrium and ventricle has a two-lead system placed in the heart—one lead is placed in the right atrium, the other in the right ventricle. This type of pacemaker is called a *dual-chamber pacemaker.* An **AV sequential pacemaker** is an example of a dual-chamber pacemaker. The AV sequential pacemaker stimulates the right atrium and right ventricle sequentially (stimulating first the atrium, then the ventricle), mimicking normal cardiac physiology and thus preserving the atrial contribution to ventricular filling (atrial kick) (Figure 8-3).

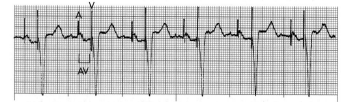

FIGURE **8-3** AV sequential pacing. *A,* atrial pacing; *V,* ventricular pacing; *AV,* AV interval.

The dual-chamber pacemaker may also be called a *DDD pacemaker,* indicating that both the atrium and ventricle are paced *(D),* both chambers are sensed *(D),* and the pacemaker has both a triggered and inhibited mode of response *(D).* When spontaneous atrial depolarization does not occur within a preset interval, the atrial pulse generator fires and stimulates atrial depolarization at a preset rate. The pacemaker is programmed to wait—simulating the normal delay in conduction through the AV node (the PR interval). The "artificial" or "electronic" PR interval is referred to as an *AV interval.* If spontaneous ventricular depolarization does not occur within a preset interval, the pacemaker fires and stimulates ventricular depolarization at a preset rate.

TRANSCUTANEOUS PACING (TCP)

Indications

Transcutaneous pacing is recommended as the initial pacing method of choice in emergency cardiac care because it is effective, quick, safe, and is the least invasive pacing technique currently available.

TCP is indicated for significant bradycardias unresponsive to atropine therapy or when atropine is not immediately available. TCP may be used as a "bridge" until transvenous pacing can be accomplished or the cause of the bradydysrhythmia is reversed (as in cases of drug overdose or hyperkalemia). TCP may be considered in asystolic cardiac arrest (less than 10 minutes in duration) and witnessed asystolic arrest.

Technique

Transcutaneous pacing involves attaching two large pacing electrodes (approximately 8 to 10 cm in diameter) to the skin surface of the patient's outer chest wall. The pacing pads used during TCP function as a bipolar pacing system. The electrical signal exits from the negative terminal on the machine (and subsequently the negative electrode) and passes through the chest wall to the heart. Depolarization of the myocardium requires an electric current strong enough to overcome the resistance of the chest wall.

The anterior (negative) chest electrode is placed to the left of the sternum, halfway between the xiphoid process and left nipple (Figure 8-4). In female patients, the anterior electrode should be positioned under the left breast. The posterior (positive) electrode is placed on the left posterior thorax directly behind the anterior electrode. The electrodes should fit completely on the patient's torso, have a minimum of 1 to 2 inches of space between electrodes, and should not overlap bony prominences of the sternum, spine, or scapula.

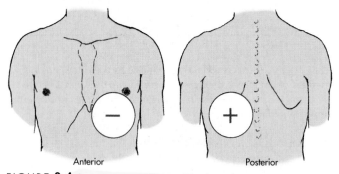

FIGURE 8-4 Anterior-posterior positioning of transcutaneous electrodes.

Studies have evaluated the importance of electrode positioning during TCP and found that, in normal volunteers, electrode placement was not crucial if the anterior electrode was of negative polarity.[13] However, electrode placement may be more significant in the critically ill patient.

If the anterior-posterior electrode position is contraindicated, the anterior-lateral position may be used. The anterior (negative) electrode is placed on the left anterior thorax, just lateral to the left nipple in the midaxillary line. The posterior (positive) electrode is placed on the right anterior upper thorax in the subclavicular area (Figure 8-5).

TCP is initiated by connecting the patient to an ECG monitor, obtaining a rhythm strip, and verifying the presence of a paceable rhythm. The pacing cable should be connected to the adhesive electrodes on the patient and to the pulse generator. After turning on the power to the pulse generator, the pacing rate should be set. In a patient with a pulse, the rate is generally set at a non-bradycardic rate between 60 and 80 beats/min. In an asystolic patient, the rate is typically set between 80 and 100 beats/min.

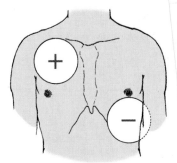

FIGURE **8-5** Anterior-lateral positioning of transcuta
electrodes.

After the rate has been regulated, the stimulating cur
put or milliamperes) is set. In a patient with a pulse, t
is increased slowly but steadily until capture is achiev
Sedation or analgesia may be needed to minimize the
fort associated with this procedure (common with cur
50 mA or more). For the asystolic patient, it is reasonable to set
the current to maximal output and then decrease the output if
capture is achieved.

Documentation should include the date and time pacing was
initiated (including baseline and pacing rhythm strips), the current required to obtain capture, the pacing rate selected, the
patient's responses to electrical and mechanical capture, medications administered during the procedure, and the date and
time pacing was terminated.

Limitations of TCP

The primary limitation of TCP is patient discomfort that is pro-
portional to the intensity of skeletal muscle contraction and the
direct electrical stimulation of cutaneous nerves. The degree of
discomfort varies with the device used and the stimulating

current required to achieve capture. Increased chest wall muscle mass, chronic obstructive pulmonary disease (COPD), or pleural effusions may require increased stimulating current.[6]

PACEMAKER MALFUNCTION

Failure to Pace

Failure to pace is a pacemaker malfunction that occurs when the pacemaker fails to deliver an electrical stimulus or when it fails to deliver the correct number of electrical stimulations per minute. Failure to pace is recognized on the ECG as an absence of pacemaker spikes (even though the patient's intrinsic rate is less than that of the pacemaker) and a return of the underlying rhythm for which the pacemaker was implanted. Patient signs and symptoms may include syncope, chest pain, bradycardia, and hypotension.

Causes of failure to pace include battery failure, fracture of the pacing lead wire, displacement of the electrode tip, pulse generator failure, a broken or loose connection between the pacing lead and the pulse generator, electromagnetic interference, and/or the sensitivity setting set too high.

Treatment may include adjusting the sensitivity setting, replacing the pulse generator battery, replacing the pacing lead, replacing the pulse generator unit, tightening connections between the pacing lead and pulse generator, performing an electrical check, and/or removing the source of electromagnetic interference.

Failure to Capture

Capture is successful depolarization of the atria and/or ventricles by an artificial pacemaker and is obtained after the pacemaker electrode is properly positioned in the heart. Failure to capture is the inability of the pacemaker stimulus to depolarize the myocardium and is recognized on the ECG by visible pacemaker spikes not followed by P waves (if the electrode is located in the atrium) or QRS complexes (if the electrode is located in

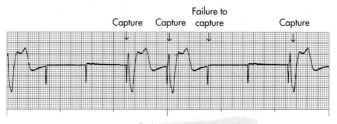

FIGURE **8-6** Failure to capture.

the right ventricle) (Figure 8-6). Patient signs and symptoms may include fatigue, bradycardia, and hypotension.

Causes of failure to capture include battery failure, fracture of the pacing lead wire, displacement of pacing lead wire (common cause), perforation of the myocardium by a lead wire, edema or scar tissue formation at the electrode tip, output energy (mA) set too low (common cause), and/or increased stimulation threshold because of medications, electrolyte imbalance, or increased fibrin formation on the catheter tip.

Treatment may include repositioning the patient, slowly increasing the output setting (mA) until capture occurs or the maximum setting is reached, replacing the pulse generator battery, replacing or repositioning of the pacing lead, or surgery.

Failure to Sense (Undersensing)

Sensitivity is the extent to which a pacemaker recognizes intrinsic electrical activity. Failure to sense occurs when the pacemaker fails to recognize spontaneous myocardial depolarization (Figure 8-7). This pacemaker malfunction is recognized on the ECG by pacemaker spikes that follow too closely behind the patient's QRS complexes (earlier than the programmed escape interval). Because pacemaker spikes occur when they should not, this type of pacemaker malfunction may result in pacemaker spikes that fall on T waves (R-on-T phenomenon) and/or

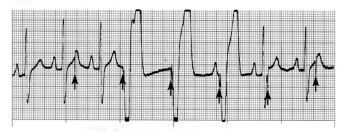

FIGURE **8-7** Failure to sense.

competition between the pacemaker and the patient's own cardiac rhythm. The patient may complain of palpitations or skipped beats. R-on-T phenomenon may precipitate VT or VF.

Causes of failure to sense include battery failure, fracture of pacing lead wire, displacement of the electrode tip (most common cause), decreased P wave or QRS voltage, circuitry dysfunction (generator unable to process QRS signal), increased sensing threshold from edema or fibrosis at the electrode tip, antidysrhythmic medications, severe electrolyte disturbances, and myocardial perforation.

Treatment may include increasing the sensitivity setting, replacing the pulse generator battery, and/or replacing or repositioning the pacing lead.

Oversensing

Oversensing is a pacemaker malfunction that results from inappropriate sensing of extraneous electrical signals. Atrial sensing pacemakers may inappropriately sense ventricular activity; ventricular sensing pacemakers may misidentify a tall, peaked intrinsic T wave as a QRS complex. Oversensing is recognized on the ECG as pacemaker spikes at a rate slower than the pacemaker's preset rate (paced QRS complexes that come later than the pacemaker's preset escape interval) or no paced beats even though the pacemaker's preset rate is greater than the patient's intrinsic rate.

The patient with a pacemaker should avoid strong electromagnetic fields such as those associated with arc welding equipment or a magnetic resonance imaging (MRI) machine. Treatment includes adjustment of the pacemaker's sensitivity setting or possible insertion of a bipolar lead if oversensing is caused by unipolar lead dysfunction.

PACEMAKER COMPLICATIONS

Complications of Transcutaneous Pacing

Complications of transcutaneous pacing include pain from electrical stimulation of the skin and muscles, failure to recognize that the pacemaker is not capturing, and failure to recognize the presence of underlying treatable VF. Tissue damage, including third-degree burns, has been reported in pediatric patients with improper or prolonged transcutaneous pacing. Prolonged pacing has been associated with pacing threshold changes, leading to capture failure.

Complications of Temporary Transvenous Pacing

Complications of temporary transvenous pacing include bleeding, infection, pneumothorax, cardiac dysrhythmias, myocardial infarction, lead displacement, fracture of the pacing lead, hematoma at the insertion site, perforation of the right ventricle with or without pericardial tamponade, and perforation of the inferior vena cava, pulmonary artery, or coronary arteries because of improper placement of the pacing lead.

Complications of Permanent Pacing

Complications of permanent pacing associated with the implantation procedure include bleeding, local tissue reaction, pneumothorax, cardiac dysrhythmias, air embolism, and thrombosis. Long-term complications of permanent pacing may include infection, electrode displacement, congestive heart failure, fracture of the pacing lead, pacemaker-induced dysrhythmias, externalization of the pacemaker generator, and perforation of the right ventricle with or without pericardial tamponade.

ANALYZING PACEMAKER FUNCTION ON THE ECG

Identify the Intrinsic Rate and Rhythm

- Are P waves present? At what rate?
- Are QRS complexes present? At what rate?

Is There Evidence of Paced Activity?

- If paced atrial activity is present, evaluate the paced interval.
- Using calipers or paper, measure the distance between two consecutively paced atrial beats.
- Determine the rate and regularity of the paced interval.
- If paced ventricular activity is present, evaluate the paced interval.
- Using calipers or paper, measure the distance between two consecutively paced ventricular beats.
- Determine the rate and regularity of the paced interval.

Evaluate the Escape Interval

- Compare the escape interval to the paced interval measured earlier. The paced interval and escape interval should measure the same.

Analyze the Rhythm Strip

- Analyze the rhythm strip for failure to capture, failure to sense, oversensing, and failure to pace.

CHAPTER **9**

Introduction
to the 12-Lead ECG

INTRODUCTION TO THE 12-LEAD ECG

A standard 12-lead ECG provides views of the heart in both the
frontal and horizontal planes and views the surfaces of the left
ventricle from 12 different angles. Multiple views of the heart
can provide useful information, including recognition of bundle
branch blocks; identification of ST segment and T wave changes
associated with myocardial ischemia, injury, and infarction; and
identification of ECG changes associated with certain medications and electrolyte imbalances.

VECTORS

Leads have a negative (−) and positive (+) electrode (pole) that
senses the magnitude and direction of the electrical force
caused by the spread of waves of depolarization and repolarization throughout the myocardium. A **vector (arrow)** is a symbol
representing this force. Leads that face the tip or point of a vector record a positive deflection on ECG paper.

131

A **mean vector** identifies the average of depolarization waves in one portion of the heart. The **mean P vector** represents the average magnitude and direction of both right and left atrial depolarization. The **mean QRS vector** represents the average magnitude and direction of both right and left ventricular depolarization. The average direction of a mean vector is called the **mean axis** and is only identified in the frontal plane. An imaginary line joining the positive and negative electrodes of a lead is called the **axis** of the lead. **Electrical axis** refers to determining the direction (or angle in degrees) in which the main vector of depolarization is pointed.

Axis

During normal ventricular depolarization, the left side of the interventricular septum is stimulated first. The electrical impulse then traverses the septum to stimulate the right side. The left and right ventricles are then depolarized simultaneously. Because the left ventricle is considerably larger than the right, right ventricular depolarization forces are overshadowed on the ECG. As a result, the mean QRS vector points down (inferior) and to the left.

The axes of leads I, II, and III form an equilateral triangle with the heart at the center (Einthoven's triangle). If the augmented limb leads are added to this configuration and the axes of the six leads moved in a way in which they bisect each other, the result is the **hexaxial reference system.**

The hexaxial reference system represents all of the frontal plane (limb) leads with the heart in the center and is the means used to express the location of the frontal plane axis. This system forms a 360-degree circle surrounding the heart. The positive end of lead I is designated at 0 degrees. The six frontal plane leads divide the circle into segments, each representing 30 degrees. All degrees in the upper hemisphere are labeled as negative degrees, and all degrees in the lower hemisphere are labeled as positive degrees. The mean QRS vector (normal electrical axis) lies between 0 and +90 degrees.

Current flow to the right of normal is called **right axis deviation** (+90 to +180 degrees). Current flow to the left of normal is called **left axis deviation** (−1 to −90 degrees). Current flow in the direction opposite of normal is called **indeterminate, "no man's land," northwest** or **extreme right axis deviation** (−91 to −179 degrees).

In the hexaxial reference system, the axes of some leads are perpendicular to each other. Lead I is perpendicular to lead aVF. Lead II is perpendicular to aVl, and lead III is perpendicular to lead aVR. If the electrical force moves toward a positive electrode, a positive (upright) deflection will be recorded. If the electrical force moves away from a positive electrode, a negative (downward) deflection will be recorded. If the electrical force is parallel to a given lead, the largest deflection in that lead will be recorded. Whether the deflection is positive or negative depends on whether the electrical force moves toward or away from the positive electrode. If the electrical force is perpendicular to a lead axis, the resulting ECG complex will be small or biphasic in that lead.

Leads I and aVF divide the heart into four quadrants. These two leads can be used to quickly estimate electrical axis. In leads I and aVF, the QRS complex is normally positive. If the QRS complex in either or both of these leads is negative, axis deviation is present (Table 9-1).

Right axis deviation may be a normal variant, particularly in the young and in thin individuals. Other causes of right axis deviation include mechanical shifts associated with inspiration or emphysema, right ventricular hypertrophy, dextrocardia, and left posterior hemiblock.

Left axis deviation may be a normal variant, particularly in older individuals and obesity. Other causes of left axis deviation

TABLE 9-1	Two-Lead Method of Axis Determination			
Axis	Normal	Left	Right	Indeterminate ("no man's land")
Lead I QRS direction	Positive	Positive	Negative	Negative
Lead aVF QRS direction	Positive	Negative	Positive	Negative

include mechanical shifts associated with expiration; a high diaphragm caused by pregnancy, ascites, or abdominal tumors; left anterior hemiblock, hyperkalemia, inspiration or emphysema, right ventricular hypertrophy, and dextrocardia.

Ischemia, Injury, and Infarction

The sudden occlusion of a coronary artery because of a thrombus may result in ischemia, injury, and/or necrosis of the area of the myocardium supplied by the affected artery. The area supplied by the obstructed artery goes through a characteristic sequence of events identified as "zones" of ischemia, injury, and infarction. Each zone is associated with characteristic ECG changes (Figure 9-1).

Acute coronary syndromes (ACS) is a term used to refer to patients presenting with ischemic chest pain. Acute coronary syndromes consist of three major syndromes that are related:

- Unstable angina
- Non-ST-segment elevation (non-Q-wave) myocardial infarction
- ST-segment elevation (Q-wave) myocardial infarction

These syndromes represent a continuum of a similar disease process involving a ruptured or eroded atheromatous plaque. Each syndrome is associated with specific strategies in prognosis and management.

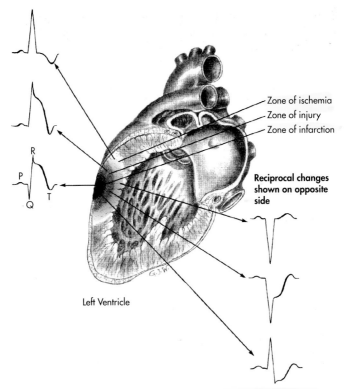

Zone of ischemia
Zone of injury
Zone of infarction

Reciprocal changes shown on opposite side

Left Ventricle

FIGURE **9-1** Zones of ischemia, injury, and infarction, showing ECG waveforms and reciprocal waveforms corresponding to each zone.

Ischemia

Myocardial ischemia results when the heart's demand for oxygen exceeds its supply from the coronary circulation. Myocardial ischemia can occur because of a decrease in myocardial oxygen supply or an increase in myocardial oxygen demand. This imbalance may be caused by decreased coronary artery blood flow because of blood vessel obstruction (atherosclerosis, vasospasm, thrombosis, embolism), decreased filling time (e.g., tachycardia), or decreased filling pressure in the coronary arteries (e.g., severe hypotension, aortic valve disease). Angina pectoris is a symptom of myocardial ischemia. The pain that accompanies angina is typically described as chest heaviness, pressure, squeezing, or constriction.

If the process is not reversed and blood flow restored, severe myocardial ischemia may lead to cellular injury and, eventually, infarction. Ischemia can quickly resolve by either reducing the oxygen needs of the heart (by resting or slowing the heart rate with medications such as beta-blockers) or increasing blood flow by dilating the coronary arteries with medications such as nitroglycerin. Myocardial ischemia delays the process of repolarization; thus, the ECG changes characteristic of ischemia include temporary changes in the ST segment and T wave. ST segment depression is suggestive of myocardial ischemia and is considered significant when the ST segment is more than 1 mm below the baseline at a point 0.04 sec (one small box) to the right of the J point (the point where the QRS ends and the ST segment begins) and is seen in two or more leads facing the same anatomic area of the heart.

If ischemia is present through the full thickness of the myocardium, a negative (inverted) T wave will be present in the leads facing the affected area of the ventricle. In leads opposite the affected area, reciprocal (mirror image) changes may be seen. If ischemia is present only in the subendocardial layer, the T wave is usually positive (upright) because the direction of repolarization is unaffected (repolarization normally occurs from epicardium to endocardium), but may be abnormally tall.[2]

T wave inversion may be seen in conditions other than myocardial ischemia, including pericarditis, bundle branch block, ventricular hypertrophy, shock, electrolyte disorders, and subarachnoid hemorrhage ("cerebral T waves").

Injury

Myocardial injury occurs when the period of ischemia is prolonged more than just a few minutes. This period is a time of severe threat to the myocardium because injured myocardial cells can live or die. If blood flow is restored to the affected area, no tissue death occurs. However, without rapid intervention, the injured area will become necrotic. Methods to restore blood flow may include administration of fibrinolytic agents, coronary angioplasty, or a coronary artery bypass graft (CABG), among others.

Injured myocardium does not function normally, affecting both muscle contraction and the conduction of electrical impulses. The injured area depolarizes incompletely and remains electrically more positive than the uninjured areas surrounding it. Thus ST segment elevation will be present in the leads facing the affected area. ST segment elevation is considered significant when the ST segment is elevated more than 1 mm above the baseline at a point 0.04 sec (one small box) to the right of the J point in the limb leads or more than 2 mm in the precordial leads, and these changes are seen in two or more leads facing the same anatomic area of the heart. In leads opposite the affected area, ST segment depression (reciprocal changes) may be seen. If injury is present only in the subendocardial layer, the ST segment is usually depressed.

Infarction

A **myocardial infarction (MI)** is the actual death of injured myocardial cells. MI occurs when there is a sudden decrease or total cessation of blood flow through a coronary artery to an area of the myocardium. This most commonly occurs because of the blockage of a coronary artery by a thrombus.

As myocardial cells die, their cell membranes break and leak substances into the bloodstream. The presence of these substances in the blood can subsequently be measured by means of blood tests to verify the presence of an infarction. These substances (called *cardiac markers* or *serum cardiac markers*) include creatine kinase (CK) MB isoforms, troponin, and myoglobin. Troponin T and troponin I are two tests that may be ordered for a patient with a suspected MI. If the level is elevated (positive test), myocardial necrosis (infarction) has almost certainly occurred. The troponin-I test appears to have better specificity than troponin-T (Table 9-2). Serum cardiac markers are useful for confirming the diagnosis of MI when patients present without ST-segment elevation, when the diagnosis may be unclear, and when physicians must distinguish patients with unstable angina from those with a non-ST-segment elevation (non-Q-wave) MI. They are also useful for confirming the diagnosis of MI for patients with ST-segment elevation.

TABLE 9-2	SERUM CARDIAC MARKERS		
	Rises	Peaks	Duration
Troponin-I	4-8 hours	12-16 hours	2 weeks
CK-MB	3-6 hours	12-24 hours	1-3 days
Myoglobin	2-4 hours	9-12 hours	1-2 days

According to the World Health Organization, the diagnosis of myocardial infarction is based on the presence of at least two of the following three criteria:

- Clinical history of ischemic-type chest discomfort
- Changes on serially obtained electrocardiographic tracings
- Rise and fall in serum cardiac markers

Whether an MI is an ST-segment elevation (Q-wave) or non-ST-segment elevation (non-Q-wave) MI depends on the degree and duration of vessel occlusion and the presence or absence of coronary collateral circulation.

Non-ST-Segment Elevation (Non-Q-Wave) Myocardial Infarction
In the acute phase of a non-ST-segment elevation (non-Q-wave) MI, the ST segment may be depressed in the leads facing the surface of the infarcted area. A non-ST-segment elevation MI can only be diagnosed if the ST segment and T wave changes are accompanied by elevations of serum cardiac markers indicative of myocardial necrosis.[2] Patients with non-ST-segment elevation acute MI are known to be at higher risk for death, reinfarction, and other morbidity than those with unstable angina. Recent data suggest the incidence of non-ST-segment elevation MI is increasing as the population of older patients with more advanced disease increases.

ST-Segment Elevation (Q-Wave) Myocardial Infarction
Most patients with ST-segment elevation will develop Q-wave MI. Only a minority of patients with ischemic chest discomfort at rest who do not have ST-segment elevation will develop Q-wave MI. A Q-wave MI is diagnosed by the development of abnormal Q waves in serial ECGs. Q-wave MIs tend to be larger than non-Q-wave MIs, reflecting more damage to the left ventricle, and are associated with a more prolonged and complete coronary thrombosis. Q waves may develop quite early in acute coronary syndromes.

With the exception of leads III and aVR, an abnormal (pathologic) Q wave is more than 0.04 sec in duration and more than 25% of the amplitude of the following R wave in that lead. An abnormal Q wave indicates the presence of dead myocardial tissue and, subsequently, a loss of electrical activity. Although abnormal Q waves can appear within hours after occlusion of a coronary artery, they more commonly appear several hours or days after the onset of signs and symptoms of an acute MI. Q waves do not reflect when an MI occurred. However, when combined with ST segment or T wave changes, their presence suggests a recent (acute) MI. Because the presence of a pathologic Q wave may take hours to develop to confirm the presence of a Q-wave MI, the patient's signs and symptoms, laboratory tests, and the presence of ST segment elevation provides the strongest evidence for the early recognition of MI.

Layout of the 12-Lead ECG

A 12-lead ECG is obtained with a 12-lead monitor that simultaneously records the leads and provides a read-out in a conventional four-column format. Each column consists of three rows. The standard limb leads are recorded in the first column, the augmented limb leads in the second column, and the precordial leads in the third and fourth columns (Table 9-3).

TABLE 9-3	Layout of the Four-Column 12-Lead ECG		
Limb leads		Precordial leads	
Standard leads	Augmented leads	V_1-V_3	V_4-V_6
Column I	Column II	Column III	Column IV
I: lateral	aVR	V_1: septum	V_4: anterior
II: inferior	aVL: lateral	V_2: septum	V_5: lateral
III: inferior	aVF: inferior	V_3: anterior	V_6: lateral

12-Lead Changes Indicating Infarction

During the evolution of an acute Q-wave MI, a typical sequence of ECG events occurs in the leads that face the infarcted area. The earliest changes include an increase in T wave amplitude. The T waves are tall, may be peaked, and are called "hyperacute" (or "tombstone") T waves. Hyperacute T waves (over 50% of preceding R wave) overlying the affected myocardium may be the first ECG sign of acute MI. They are transient, often seen within minutes or hours after the onset of chest pain, and are believed to be caused by subendocardial ischemia.[2] Hyperacute T waves are followed by ST segment elevation and then the appearance of pathologic Q waves (in Q-wave infarction) in the leads facing the affected area. The evolution of the MI continues with decreased R wave amplitude (poor R-wave progression) and T-wave inversion.

In the standard 12-lead ECG, leads II, III, and aVF "look" at tissue supplied by the right coronary artery and eight leads "look" at tissue supplied by the left coronary artery—leads I, aVL, V_1, V_2, V_3, V_4, V_5, and V_6. When evaluating the extent of infarction produced by a left coronary artery occlusion, determine how many of these leads are showing changes consistent with an acute infarction. The more of these eight leads demonstrating acute changes, the larger the infarction is presumed to be.[15]

To view the right ventricle, right precordial leads are used. Placement of right precordial leads is identical to placement of the standard precordial leads except on the right side of the chest. If time does not permit obtaining all the right precordial leads, the lead of choice is V_4R. A modification of lead V_4R (MC_4R) using a standard 3-lead system may be used to view the right ventricle. The positive electrode is placed in the fifth intercostal space, right midclavicular line. The negative electrode is placed on the left arm and the lead selector on the monitor placed in the lead III position.

Because no leads of the standard 12-lead ECG directly view the posterior wall of the left ventricle, changes in the opposite (anterior) wall of the heart can be viewed as reciprocal changes. Alternately, additional precordial leads may be used to view the heart's posterior surface. These leads are placed further left and toward the back. All of the leads are placed on the same horizontal line as V_4 to V_6. Lead V_7 is placed at the posterior axillary line. Lead V_8 is placed at the angle of the scapula (posterior scapular line), and Lead V_9 is placed over the border of spine.

LOCALIZATION OF INFARCTIONS

The left ventricle has been divided into four regions where a myocardial infarction may occur—anterior, lateral, inferior, and posterior. Figure 9-2 shows which coronary artery supplies blood to each portion of the heart, the site of infarction if one of these vessels is occluded, and the area of the heart viewed by each of the leads in a standard 12-lead ECG. A myocardial infarction may not be limited to one of the regions previously described. For example, if the precordial leads indicate ECG changes in leads V_3 and V_4, suggestive of an anterior wall MI, and diagnostic changes are also present in V_5 and V_6, the infarction would be called an *anterolateral infarction* or an *anterior infarction with lateral extension.*

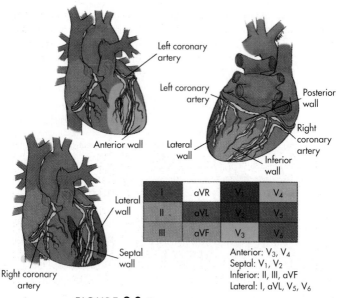

I	aVR	V₁	V₄
II	aVL	V₂	V₅
III	aVF	V₃	V₆

Anterior: V_3, V_4
Septal: V_1, V_2
Inferior: II, III, aVF
Lateral: I, aVL, V_5, V_6

FIGURE **9-2** Coronary artery anatomy.

Lateral Wall

Leads I, aVL, V_5, and V_6 view the lateral wall of the left ventricle. The lateral wall is usually supplied by the circumflex branch of the left coronary artery. Lateral wall infarctions often occur as extensions of anterior or inferior infarctions. ECG changes suggestive of MI include ST segment elevation in leads I, aVL, V_5, and V_6.

Reciprocal ST depression may be seen in V_1.

Inferior Wall

Leads II, III, and aVF view the inferior surface of the left ventricle. Reciprocal changes are observed in leads I and aVL. In most individuals, the inferior wall of the left ventricle is supplied by the posterior descending branch of the right coronary artery. ECG changes suggestive of infarction include ST segment elevation in leads II, III, and aVF (Figure 9-3).

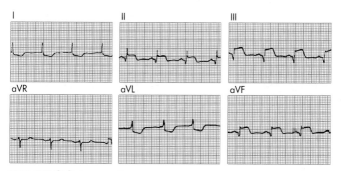

FIGURE 9-3 Acute inferior wall infarction. Note the ST segment elevation in leads II, III, and aVF and the reciprocal ST depression in leads I and aVL. Abnormal Q waves are also present in leads II, III, and aVF.

Septum

Leads V_1 and V_2 face the septal area of the left ventricle. The septum, which contains the bundle of His and bundle branches, is normally supplied by the left anterior descending artery. ECG changes suggestive of infarction include the absence of normal "septal" R waves in leads V_1 and V_2 (resulting in QS waves in these leads) (Figure 9-4); absence of normal "septal" Q waves in leads I, II, III, aVF, V_4, V_5, and V_6; and ST segment elevation with tall T waves in leads V_1 and V_2.

Anterior Wall

Leads V_3 and V_4 face the anterior wall of the left ventricle. Reciprocal changes of injury, such as ST depression, appear in leads II, III, and aVF. This area is normally supplied by the diagonal branch of the left anterior descending artery. ECG changes suggestive of infarction include ST segment elevation with tall T waves and taller than normal R waves in leads V_3 and V_4 (Figure 9-5).

Posterior Wall

The posterior wall of the left ventricle is supplied by the left circumflex coronary artery in most patients; however, in some patients it is supplied by the right coronary artery. On the standard 12-lead ECG, no leads directly view the posterior wall of the left ventricle. Changes in the opposite (anterior) wall of the heart can be viewed as reciprocal changes (Figure 9-6). A posterior wall MI usually produces tall R waves and ST segment depression in leads V_1 through V_4.

Right Ventricular Infarction

Right ventricular infarction (RVI) should be suspected when ECG changes suggesting an acute inferior wall MI (viewed in leads II, III, and aVF) are observed. When RVI is suspected, right precordial leads are used. ST segment elevation of 1 mm

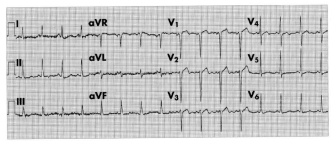

FIGURE **9-4** Septal infarction. Poor R-wave progression.

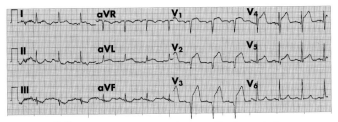

FIGURE **9-5** Extensive anterior infarction. Reciprocal changes present in leads II, III, and aVF.

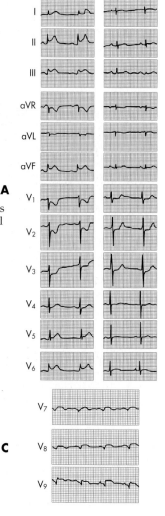

A

B

C

FIGURE **9-6** Evolutionary changes in inferior and posterior myocardial infarction (MI). **A,** Acute inferior and apical injury. **B,** At 24 hours. Note tall R wave in lead V_1 not present in **A,** suggesting posterior MI. **C,** Posterior infarction confirmed.

or more in lead V_4R has a sensitivity of 70% to 93% and a specificity of 77% to 100%[2] (Figure 9-7). A right ventricular MI
should be suspected in the patient with an inferior left ventricular MI; unexplained, persistent hypotension; clear lung fields;
and jugular venous distention (Table 9-4).

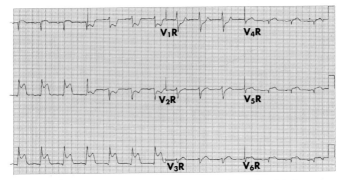

FIGURE 9-7 A 12-lead ECG obtained using the right-sided precordial leads. Inferior infarction with evidence of right ventricular
injury (V_4R).

INTRAVENTRICULAR CONDUCTION DELAYS

Intraventricular conduction delays are best identified by using
leads MCL_1, MCL_6, V_1, and/or V_6.

If a delay or block occurs in one of the bundle branches, the
ventricles will be depolarized asynchronously. The impulse
travels first down the unblocked branch and stimulates that
ventricle. Because of the block, the impulse must then travel
from cell to cell through the myocardium (rather than through
the normal conduction pathway) to stimulate the other ventricle. This means of conduction is slower than normal and the
QRS complex appears widened on the ECG. The ventricle with

TABLE **9-4**	LOCALIZATION OF A MYOCARDIAL INFARCTION		
Location of MI	Indicative changes (leads facing affected area)	Reciprocal changes (leads opposite affected area)	Affected coronary artery
Lateral	I, aVL, V_5, V_6	V_1-V_3	Left coronary artery—circumflex branch
Inferior	II, III, aVF	I, aVL	Right coronary artery—posterior descending branch
Septum	V_1, V_2	None	Left coronary artery—left anterior descending artery, septal branch
Anterior	V_3, V_4	II, III, aVF	Left coronary artery—left anterior descending artery, diagonal branch
Posterior	Not visualized	V_1, V_2, V_3, V_4	Right coronary artery or left circumflex artery
Right ventricle	V_1R-V_6R		Right coronary artery—proximal branches

the blocked, bundle branch is the last to be depolarized. A QRS measuring 0.10 to 0.12 sec is called an **incomplete** right or left bundle branch block. A QRS measuring more than 0.12 sec is called a **complete** right or left bundle branch block. If the QRS is wide but there is no BBB pattern, the term *wide QRS* or *intraventricular conduction delay* is used to describe the QRS.

The width of a QRS complex is most accurately determined when it is viewed and measured in more than one lead. The measurement should be taken from the QRS complex with the longest duration and clearest onset and end.

ECG criteria for identification of a right or left BBB are:

- A QRS duration of more than 0.12 sec (if a complete BBB)
- QRS complexes produced by supraventricular activity (i.e., the QRS complex is not a paced beat nor did it originate in the ventricles)

To determine right vs. left BBB:

- View lead V_1 or MCL_1
- Move from the J point back into the QRS complex and determine if the terminal portion (last 0.04 sec) of the QRS complex is a positive (upright) or negative (downward) deflection
- If the two criteria for bundle branch block are met and the terminal portion of the QRS is positive, a RBBB is most likely present
- If the terminal portion of the QRS is negative, a LBBB is most likely present

CHAMBER ENLARGEMENT

Enlargement of the atrial and/or ventricular chambers of the heart may occur if there is a volume or pressure overload in the heart. **Dilatation** is an increase in the diameter of a chamber of the heart caused by volume overload. Dilatation may be acute or chronic. **Hypertrophy** is an increase in the thickness of a heart chamber because of chronic pressure overload. **Enlargement** is a term that implies presence of dilatation or hypertrophy, or both.

Atrial Enlargement

Right Atrium

Enlargement of the right atrium produces an abnormally tall initial part of the P wave. The P wave is tall (2.5 mm or more in height in leads II, III, and aVF), peaked, and of normal duration. This type of P wave is called *P pulmonale* because right atrial enlargement (RAE) is usually caused by conditions that increase the work of the right atrium, such as chronic obstructive pulmonary disease with or without pulmonary hypertension, congenital heart disease, or right ventricular failure of any cause. The P wave may be biphasic in lead V_1 with a more prominent positive portion.

Left Atrium

The latter part of the P wave is prominent in left atrial enlargement (LAE). This is because the impulse starts in the right atrium where the SA node is located and chamber size is normal. The electrical impulse then travels to the left to depolarize the left atrium. The waveform inscribed on the ECG is widened (latter part of the P wave) because it takes longer to depolarize an enlarged muscle. The P wave is more than 0.11 sec in duration and often notched in leads I, II, aVL, and V_4, V_5, and V_6. The P wave may be biphasic in lead V_1 with a more prominent negative portion. LAE occurs because of conditions that increase left atrial pressure or volume overload or both. These conditions include mitral regurgitation, mitral stenosis, left ventricular failure, and systemic hypertension. Because of the frequent association of LAE with mitral valve disease, the wide, notched P wave that is usually seen is called *P mitrale*.

Ventricular Enlargement

Ventricular muscle thickens (hypertrophies) when it sustains a persistent pressure overload. Dilatation occurs because of persistent volume overload. The two often go hand in hand. Hypertrophy increases the QRS amplitude and is often associated with ST-segment depression and asymmetric T-wave inversion. The ST-segment depression and T-wave inversion pattern is called *ventricular strain* or *secondary repolarization changes*.

The amplitude (voltage) of the QRS complex can be affected by various factors, including age, body weight, and lung disease. Increased QRS amplitude may occur normally in thin-chested individuals or young adults because the chest electrodes are closer to the heart in these patients.[16]

Right Ventricle
Because the right ventricle is normally considerably smaller than the left, it must become extremely enlarged before changes are visible on the ECG. Right axis deviation is one of the earliest and most reliable findings of right ventricular hypertrophy (RVH).[16] Further, normal R-wave progression is reversed in the precordial leads, revealing taller than normal R waves and small S waves in V_1 and V_2 and deeper than normal S waves and small R waves in V_5 and V_6. Ventricular activation time (VAT) is delayed in V_1. Causes of RVH include pulmonary hypertension and chronic lung diseases, valvular heart disease, and congenital heart disease.

Left Ventricle
Recognition of left ventricular hypertrophy (LVH) on the ECG is not always obvious, and many methods to assist in its recognition have been suggested. ECG signs of LVH include deeper than normal S waves and small R waves in V_1 and V_2 and taller than normal R waves and small S waves in V_5 and V_6. If the S-wave amplitude in lead V_1 added to the R-wave amplitude in V_5 is greater than or equal to 35 mV, LVH should be suspected. Other ECG changes suggesting the presence of LVH include an R-wave amplitude in lead aVL greater than or equal to 12 mV. Evidence of delayed ventricular activation time may be visible in V_6, and secondary repolarization changes (strain pattern) are often seen in V_5 and V_6. Causes of LVH include systemic hypertension, hypertrophic cardiomyopathy, aortic stenosis, and aortic insufficiency.

ECG CHANGES ASSOCIATED WITH ELECTROLYTE DISTURBANCES

ECG changes associated with electrolyte disturbances are summarized in Table 9-5.

TABLE 9-5	ECG Changes Associated With Electrolyte Disturbances					
Medication	P wave	PR interval	QRS complex	ST segment	T wave	QT interval	Heart rate
Hypocalcemia				Long, flattened		Prolonged	
Hypercalcemia		Prolonged		Shortened		Shortened	
Hypokalemia			Widened as level decreases	Depressed	Flattened; U wave present	Prolonged	
Hyperkalemia	Disappear as level increases	Normal or prolonged	Widened as level increases	Disappears as level increases	Tall, peaked/ tented		Slows
Hypomagnesemia	Diminished voltage (amplitude)		Widened as level decreases; diminished voltage	Depressed	Flattened; U wave present	Prolonged	
Hypermagnesemia		Prolonged	Widened		Tall/elevated		

Analyzing the 12-Lead ECG

When analyzing a 12-lead ECG, it is important to use a systematic method. Findings suggestive of an acute MI are considered significant if viewed in two or more leads looking at the same area of the heart. If these findings are viewed in leads that look directly at the affected area, they are called *indicative changes*. If findings are observed in leads opposite the affected area, they are called *reciprocal changes*.

- Rate: atrial and ventricular
- Rhythm: atrial and ventricular
- Intervals: PR interval, QRS duration, QT interval
- Waveforms: P waves, Q waves, R waves (R-wave progression), T waves, U waves
- ST segment: elevation, depression
- Axis
- Hypertrophy/chamber enlargement
- Myocardial ischemia, injury, infarction
- Effects of medications and electrolyte imbalances

References

1. Taylor G: *150 practice ECGs: interpretation and board review,* Cambridge, 1997, Blackwell Science.
2. Chou T, Knilans TK: *Electrocardiography in clinical practice: adult and pediatric,* Philadelphia, 1996, WB Saunders.
3. Wagner GS: *Marriott's practical electrocardiography,* ed 9, Baltimore, 1994, Williams & Wilkins.
4. Weil MH, Tang W, editors: *CPR: resuscitation of the arrested heart,* Philadelphia, 1999, WB Saunders.
5. Murphy JG: *Mayo clinical cardiology review,* ed 2, Philadelphia, 2000, Lippincott, Williams & Wilkins.
6. Crawford MV, Spence MI: *Common sense approach to coronary care,* ed 6, St Louis, 1995, Mosby.
7. Woods SL, Sivarajan Froelicher ES, Motzer SA: *Cardiac nursing,* ed 4, Philadelphia, 2000, Lippincott, Williams & Wilkins.
8. Padrid PJ, Kowey PR, editors: *Cardiac arrhythmia: mechanisms, diagnosis, and management,* Baltimore, 1995, Williams & Wilkins.
9. Goldberger AL: *Clinica electrocardiography: a simplified approach,* ed 6, St Louis, 1999, Mosby.
10. Goldman L, Braunwald E: *Primary cardiology,* Philadelphia, 1998, WB Saunders.
11. Paradis NA, Halperin HR, Nowak RM, editors: *Cardiac arrest: the science and practice of resuscitation medicine,* Baltimore, 1996, Williams & Wilkins.

12. Barold SS: Indications for permanent cardiac pacing in first-degree AV block: class I, II, or III? *PACE Pacing Clin Electrophysiol* 19:747-751, 1996.
13. Falk RH, Ngai S: External cardiac pacing: influence of electrode placement, *Crit Care Med* 14:11, 1986.
14. Gibler WB: *Emergency cardiac care,* St Louis, 1994, Mosby.
15. Phalen T: *The 12-lead ECG in acute myocardial infarction,* St Louis, 1996, Mosby.

Glossary

A wave: Atrial-paced event; the atrial stimulus or the point in the intrinsic atrial depolarization (P wave) at which atrial sensing occurs; analogous to the P wave of intrinsic waveforms

AA interval: Interval between two consecutive atrial stimuli, with or without an interceding ventricular event; analogous to the P-P interval of intrinsic waveforms

AV interval: In dual-chamber pacing, the length of time between an atrial-sensed or atrial-paced event and the delivery of a ventricular pacing stimulus; analogous to the P-R interval of intrinsic waveforms

aberrant: Abnormal

absolute refractory period: Corresponds with the onset of the QRS complex to approximately the peak of the T wave; cardiac cells cannot be stimulated to conduct an electrical impulse no matter how strong the stimulus

accelerated idioventricular rhythm (AIVR): Dysrhythmia originating in the ventricles with a rate between 40 and 100 beats/min

accelerated junctional rhythm: Dysrhythmia originating in the AV junction with a rate between 60 and 100 beats/min

accessory pathway: Extra muscle bundle consisting of working myocardial tissue that forms a connection between the atria and ventricles outside the normal conduction system

action potential: Reflection of the difference in the concentration of ions across a cell membrane at any given time

acute coronary syndromes: Term used to refer to patients presenting with ischemic chest pain. Acute coronary syndromes consist of three major syndromes—unstable angina, non-ST-segment elevation MI, and ST-segment elevation MI

adrenergic: Having the characteristics of the sympathetic division of the autonomic nervous system

afterload: Pressure or resistance against which the ventricles must pump to eject blood

agonal rhythm: Dysrhythmia similar in appearance to an idioventricular rhythm but occurring at a rate of less than 20 beats/min; dying heart

amplitude: Height (voltage) of a waveform on the ECG

angina: Chest pain of sudden onset that may occur because the increased oxygen demand of the heart temporarily exceeds the blood supply

aortic valve: Semilunar valve located between the left ventricle and aorta

apex of the heart: Lower portion of the heart; tip of the ventricles (approximately the level of the fifth left intercostal space); points leftward, downward, and forward

arrhythmia: Term often used interchangeably with *dysrhythmia;* any disturbance or abnormality in a normal rhythmic pattern; any cardiac rhythm other than a sinus rhythm

artifact: Distortion of an ECG tracing by electrical activity that is noncardiac in origin (e.g., electrical interference, poor electrical conduction, patient movement)

asynchronous pacemaker: Fixed-rate pacemaker that continuously discharges at a preset rate regardless of the patient's intrinsic activity

asystole: Absence of cardiac electrical activity viewed as a straight (isoelectric) line on the ECG

atria: Two upper chambers of the heart (singular = atrium)

atrial kick: Blood pushed into the ventricles because of atrial contraction

atrial pacing: Pacing system with a lead attached to the right atrium, designed to correct abnormalities in the SA node (sick sinus syndrome)

atrial tachycardia: Three or more sequential premature atrial complexes (PACs) occurring at a rate of more than 100 beats/min

atrioventricular (AV) valve: Valve located between each atrium and ventricle; the tricuspid separates the right atrium from the right ventricle, the mitral (bicuspid) separates the left atrium from the left ventricle

augmented lead: Leads aVR, aVL, and aVF; these leads record the difference in electrical potential at one location relative to zero potential rather than relative to the electrical potential of another extremity as in the bipolar leads

automatic interval: Period, expressed in milliseconds, between two consecutively paced events in the same cardiac chamber without an intervening sensed event (e.g., AA interval, VV interval). Also known as the *demand interval, basic interval,* or *pacing interval.*

automaticity: Ability of cardiac pacemaker cells to spontaneously initiate an electrical impulse without being stimulated from another source (such as a nerve)

AV dissociation: Any dysrhythmia in which the atria and ventricles beat independently (e.g., ventricular tachycardia, complete AV block)

AV junction: AV node and the bundle of His

AV node: Specialized cells located in the lower portion of the right atrium; delays the electrical impulse in order to allow the atria to contract and complete filling of the ventricles

AV sequential pacemaker: Type of dual-chamber pacemaker that stimulates first the atrium, then the ventricle, mimicking normal cardiac physiology

axis: Imaginary line joining the positive and negative electrodes of a lead

base of the heart: Top of the heart located at approximately the level of the second intercostal space

baseline: Straight line recorded on ECG graph paper when no electrical activity is detected

base rate: Rate at which the pulse generator of a pacemaker paces when no intrinsic activity is detected; expressed in pulse/min (ppm)

BBB: Bundle branch block

bifascicular block: Block in two divisions of the bundle branches. Although this term may be used to describe a block in both the anterior and posterior branches of the left bundle branch, it is more commonly used to describe a combination of a right bundle branch block and either a left anterior fascicular block (LAFB) or a left posterior fascicular block (LPFB)

bigeminy: Dysrhythmia in which every other beat is a premature ectopic beat

bipolar limb lead: ECG lead consisting of a positive and negative electrode; a pacing lead with two electrical poles that are external from the pulse generator. The negative pole is located at the extreme distal tip of the pacing lead. The positive pole is located several millimeters proximal to the negative electrode. The stimulating pulse is delivered through the negative electrode.

biphasic: Waveform that is partly positive and partly negative

blocked PAC (nonconducted PAC): Premature atrial complex that is not followed by a QRS complex

blood pressure: Force exerted by the circulating blood volume on the walls of the arteries. Blood pressure is equal to cardiac output times peripheral resistance.

bpm: Beats/min; the abbreviation bpm usually refers to an intrinsic heart rate, while pulse/min (ppm) usually refers to a paced rate

bradycardia: Heart rate slower than 60 beats/min (brady = slow)

bundle branch block: Abnormal conduction of an electrical impulse through either the right or left bundle branches

bundle of His: Cardiac fibers located in the upper portion of the interventricular septum; connects the AV node with the two bundle branches

burst: Three or more sequential ectopic beats; also referred to as a "salvo" or "run"

bypass tract: Term used when one end of an accessory pathway is attached to normal conductive tissue

calibration: Regulation of an ECG machine's stylus sensitivity so that a 1 mV electrical signal will produce a deflection measuring exactly 10 mm

capacitor: Device that can store an electrical charge

capture: Ability of a pacing stimulus to successfully depolarize the cardiac chamber that is being paced. With one-to-one capture, each pacing stimulus results in depolarization of the appropriate chamber.

cardiac arrest: Clinical death characterized by cessation of pulse and respiration

cardiac cycle: Period from the beginning of one heart beat to the beginning of the next one; normally consisting of PQRST waves, complexes, and intervals

cardiac index: Measure of a patient's cardiac output per square meter of body surface area (BSA)

cardiac output: Amount of blood pumped into the aorta each minute by the heart

carotid sinus pressure: Type of vagal maneuver in which pressure is applied to the carotid sinus for a brief period to slow conduction through the AV node

catecholamines: Natural chemicals produced by the body that have sympathetic actions (epinephrine, norepinephrine, dopamine)

cholinergic: Having the characteristics of the parasympathetic division of the autonomic nervous system

chordae tendineae: Thin strands of fibrous connective tissue that extend from the AV valves to the papillary muscles and prevent the AV valves from bulging back into the atria during ventricular systole (contraction)

chronotropism: Refers to a change in heart rate. Positive chronotropic effect refers to an increase in heart rate. Negative chronotropic effect refers to a decrease in heart rate

circumflex artery: Division of the left coronary artery

coarse ventricular fibrillation: Ventricular fibrillation with fibrillatory waves greater than 3 mm in height

compensatory pause: Pause is termed *compensatory* (or *complete)* if the normal beat following a premature complex occurs when expected

complex: Several waveforms

conductivity: Ability of a cardiac cell to receive an electrical stimulus and conduct that impulse to an adjacent cardiac cell

contractility: Ability of cardiac cells to shorten, causing cardiac muscle contraction in response to an electrical stimulus

coronary sinus: Outlet that drains five coronary veins into the right atrium

couplet: Two consecutive premature complexes

coupling interval: Interval between an ectopic beat and the preceding beat of the underlying rhythm

cycle length: Term used for the period between any one type of event and the next event of the same type, usually expressed in milliseconds

defibrillation: Therapeutic use of electric current to terminate lethal cardiac dysrhythmias

delta wave: Slurring of the beginning portion of the QRS complex, caused by preexcitation

demand interval: Period, expressed in milliseconds, between two consecutively paced events in the same cardiac chamber without an intervening sensed event (e.g., AA interval, VV interval). Also known as the *basic interval* or *pacing interval*

demand pacemaker: Synchronous pacemaker that discharges only when the patient's heart rate drops below the preset rate for the pacemaker

depolarization: Movement of ions across a cell membrane, causing the inside of the cell to become more positive; an electrical event expected to result in contraction

dextrocardia: Location of the heart in the right thorax because of a congenital defect or displacement by disease

diastole: Phase of the cardiac cycle in which the atria and ventricles relax between contractions and blood enters these chambers. When the term is used without reference to a specific chamber of the heart, the term implies ventricular diastole

dilatation: Increase in the diameter of a chamber of the heart because of volume overload

diphasic: Waveform that is partly positive and partly negative

dual-chamber pacemaker: Pacemaker that stimulates the atrium and ventricle

dyspnea: Shortness of breath or difficulty breathing

dysrhythmia: Any disturbance or abnormality in a normal rhythmic pattern; any cardiac rhythm other than a sinus rhythm

ectopic: Impulse(s) originating from a source other than the sinoatrial node

electrical axis: Direction (or angle in degrees) in which the main vector of depolarization is pointed

electrodes: Adhesive pads that contain a conductive gel, applied at specific locations on the patient's chest wall and extremities and connected by means of cables to an electrocardiograph

electrolyte: Element or compound that, when melted or dissolved in water or another solvent, breaks into ions (atoms able to carry an electric charge)

endocardium: Innermost layer of the heart that lines the inside of the myocardium and covers the heart valves

enhanced automaticity: Abnormal condition in which cardiac cells not normally associated with the property of automaticity begin to depolarize spontaneously or when escape pacemaker sites increase their firing rate beyond that considered normal

enlargement: Term that implies the presence of dilatation or hypertrophy or both

epicardium: Also known as the *visceral pericardium;* the external layer of the heart wall that covers the heart muscle

escape: Term used when the sinus node slows down or fails to initiate depolarization and a lower pacemaker site spontaneously produces electrical impulses, assuming responsibility for pacing the heart

escape interval: Time measured between a sensed cardiac event and the next pacemaker output

excitability: Ability of cardiac muscle cells to respond to an outside stimulus

extrasystole: Premature complex

extreme right axis deviation: Current flow in the direction opposite of normal (-91 to -179 degrees)

f waves: Fibrillation waves; irregularly shaped atrial waves associated with atrial fibrillation, occurring at a rate of 400 to 600 beats/min

F waves: Flutter waves; atrial waves associated with atrial flutter, usually shaped like the teeth of a saw or a picket fence

fascicle: Small bundle of nerve fibers

fine ventricular fibrillation: Ventricular fibrillation with fibrillatory waves less than 3 mm in height

fixed-rate pacemaker: Asynchronous pacemaker that continuously discharges at a preset rate regardless of the patient's heart rate

fusion beat: Beat that occurs because of simultaneous activation of one cardiac chamber by two sites (foci); in pacing, the ECG waveform that results when an intrinsic depolarization and a pacing stimulus occur simultaneously and both contribute to depolarization of that cardiac chamber

great vessels: Pulmonary arteries, pulmonary veins, aorta, superior, and inferior vena cavae

ground electrode: Third ECG electrode (the first and second are the positive and negative electrodes), which minimizes electrical activity from other sources

His-Purkinje system: Portion of the conduction system consisting of the bundle of His, bundle branches, and Purkinje fibers

hypertrophy: Increase in the thickness of a heart chamber because of chronic pressure overload

hysteresis: Programmable feature in some demand pacemakers that allows programming of a longer escape interval between the intrinsic complex and the first paced event

incomplete compensatory pause: Pause is termed *incomplete* (or *noncompensatory*) if the normal beat following the premature complex occurs before it was expected

indeterminate axis deviation: Current flow in the direction opposite of normal (-91 to -179 degrees)

infarction: Necrosis of tissue because of an inadequate blood supply

inherent: Natural, intrinsic

inhibition: Pacemaker response in which the output pulse is suppressed (inhibited) when an intrinsic event is sensed

inotropic effect: Refers to a change in myocardial contractility

interpolated PVC: PVC that occurs between two normal QRS complexes and does not interrupt the underlying rhythm

interval: Waveform and a segment; in pacing, the period, measured in milliseconds, between any two designated cardiac events

intrinsic rate: Rate at which a pacemaker of the heart normally generates impulses

ion: Electrically charged particle

ischemia: Decreased supply of oxygenated blood to a body part or organ

isoelectric line: Absence of electrical activity observed on the ECG as a straight line

J point: Point where the QRS complex and ST segment meet

junctional escape rhythm: Dysrhythmia originating in the AV junction that occurs when the sinoatrial node fails to pace the heart or AV conduction fails; characterized by a rhythmic rate of 40 to 60 beats/min

junctional tachycardia: Dysrhythmia originating in the AV junction with a ventricular response greater than 100 beats/min

KVO: Abbreviation meaning, "keep the vein open." Also known as *TKO*, "to keep open"

LBBB: Left bundle branch block

lead: Electrical connection attached to the body to record electrical activity

left anterior descending artery: Division of the left coronary artery

left axis deviation: Current flow to the left of normal (-1 to -90 degrees)

Lown-Ganong-Levine syndrome (LGL): Type of preexcitation syndrome in which part or all of the AV conduction system is bypassed by an abnormal AV connection from the atrial muscle to the bundle of His; characterized by a short PR interval (usually less than 0.12 sec) and a normal QRS duration

mean axis: Average direction of a mean vector; the mean axis is only identified in the frontal plane

mean vector: Average of depolarization waves in one portion of the heart

mean P vector: Average magnitude and direction of both right and left atrial depolarization

mean QRS vector: Average magnitude and direction of both right and left ventricular depolarization

mediastinum: Located in the middle of the thoracic cavity; contains the heart, great vessels, trachea, and esophagus, among other structures; extends from the sternum to the vertebral column

membrane potential: Difference in electrical charge across the cell membrane

milliampere (mA): Unit of measure of electrical current needed to elicit depolarization of the myocardium

monofascicular block: Block in only one of the fascicles of the bundle branches

monomorphic: Having the same shape

multiformed atrial rhythm: Cardiac dysrhythmia that occurs because of impulses originating from various sites, including the sinoatrial node, the atria, and/or the AV junction; requires at least three different P waves, seen in the same lead, for proper diagnosis

mV: Millivolt

myocardial cells: Working cells of the myocardium that contain contractile filaments and form the muscular layer of the atrial walls and the thicker muscular layer of the ventricular walls

myocardial infarction (MI): Necrosis of some mass of the heart muscle caused by an inadequate blood supply

myocardium: Middle and thickest layer of the heart; contains the cardiac muscle fibers that cause contraction of the heart and contains the conduction system and blood supply

myofibril: Slender striated strand of muscle tissue

nodal: Term formerly used for junctional beats or rhythms

no man's land (extreme right axis deviation): Current flow in the direction opposite of normal (−91 to −179 degrees)

noncompensatory pause: Pause is termed *noncompensatory* (or *incomplete*) if the normal beat following the premature complex occurs before it was expected

nonconducted PAC (blocked PAC): Premature atrial complex that is not followed by a QRS complex

nontransmural infarction: Myocardial infarction that is classified as either **subendocardial,** involving the endocardium and the myocardium, or **subepicardial,** involving the myocardium and the epicardium

output: Electrical stimulus delivered by a pacemaker's pulse generator, usually defined in terms of pulse amplitude (volts) and pulse width (milliseconds)

overdrive pacing: Pacing the heart at a rate faster than the rate of the tachycardia

PAC: Premature atrial complex

pacing interval: Period, expressed in milliseconds, between two consecutively paced events in the same cardiac chamber without an intervening sensed event (e.g., AA interval, VV interval). Also known as the *demand interval* or *basic interval.*

pacemaker: Artificial pulse generator that delivers an electrical current to the heart to stimulate depolarization

pacemaker cells: Specialized cells of the heart's electrical conduction system capable of spontaneously generating and conducting electrical impulses

pacemaker generator (pulse generator): Power source that houses the battery and controls for regulating a pacemaker

pacemaker spike: Vertical line on the ECG that indicates the pacemaker has discharged

pacemaker syndrome: Adverse clinical signs and symptoms that limit a patient's everyday functioning, occurring in the setting of an electrically normal pacing system. Pacemaker syndrome is most commonly associated with a loss of AV synchrony (e.g., VVI pacing) but may also occur because of an inappropriate AV interval or inappropriate rate modulation

pacing system analyzer (PSA): External testing and measuring device capable of pacing the heart during pacemaker implantation and used to determine appropriate pulse generator settings for the individual patient (e.g., pacing threshold, lead impedance, pulse amplitude)

paired beats: Two consecutive premature complexes

papillary muscles: Projections of myocardium found on the ventricular walls; during ventricular contraction the papillary muscles contract, pulling on the chordae tendineae, preventing inversion of the AV valves into the atria

parameter: Value that can be measured and sometimes changed, either indirectly or directly. In pacing, parameter refers to a value that influences the function of the pacemaker (e.g., sensitivity, amplitude, mode)

paroxysmal: Term used to describe the sudden onset or cessation of a dysrhythmia

paroxysmal atrial tachycardia (PAT): Atrial tachycardia that starts or ends suddenly

paroxysmal supraventricular tachycardia (PSVT): Term used to describe supraventricular tachycardia that starts and ends suddenly

pericardium: Protective sac that surrounds the heart

peripheral resistance: Resistance to the flow of blood, determined by blood vessel diameter and the tone of the vascular musculature

PJC: Premature junctional complex

polarized state: Period of time following repolarization of a myocardial cell (also called the *resting state*) when the outside of the cell is positive and the interior of the cell is negative

polymorphic: Varying in shape

ppm: Abbreviation for pulses/min; usually refers to a paced rate, while beats/min (bpm) refers to an intrinsic heart rate

preexcitation: Term used to describe rhythms that originate from above the ventricles but in which the impulse travels via a pathway other than the AV node and bundle of His; thus, the supraventricular impulse excites the ventricles earlier than normal

preload: Force exerted by the blood on the walls of the ventricles at the end of diastole

premature complex: Early beat occurring before the next expected beat

prophylaxis: Preventive treatment

pulse generator: Power source that houses the battery and controls for regulating a pacemaker

pulseless electrical activity (PEA): Organized electrical activity observed on a cardiac monitor (other than VT or VF) without a palpable pulse

Purkinje fibers: Elaborate web of fibers distributed throughout the ventricular myocardium

PVC: Premature ventricular complex

quadrigeminy: Dysrhythmia in which every fourth beat is a premature ectopic beat

R wave: On an EGG, the first positive deflection in the QRS complex, representing ventricular depolarization. In pacing, R wave refers to the entire QRS complex, denoting an intrinsic ventricular event

rate modulation: Ability of a pacemaker to increase the pacing rate in response to physical activity or metabolic demand. Some type of physiologic sensor is used by the pacemaker to determine the need for an increased pacing rate. Also called *rate adaptation* or *rate response.*

RBBB: Right bundle branch block

reentry: Propagation of an impulse through tissue already activated by that same impulse

refractoriness: Term used to describe the extent to which a cell is able to respond to a stimulus.

relative refractory period: Corresponds with the downslope of the T wave; cardiac cells can be stimulated to depolarize if the stimulus is strong enough

repolarization: Movement of ions across a cell membrane in which the inside of the cell is restored to its negative charge

retrograde: Moving backward; moving in the opposite direction to that which is considered normal

right axis deviation: Current flow to the right of normal (+90 to +180 degrees)

run: Three or more sequential ectopic beats; also referred to as a "salvo" or "burst"

RV interval: Period from the intrinsic ventricular event and the ventricular-paced event that follows; the pacemaker's escape interval

salvo: Three or more sequential ectopic beats; also referred to as a "run" or "burst"

sarcolemma: Membrane that covers smooth, striated, and cardiac muscle fibers

sarcomere: Smallest functional unit of a myofibril

sarcoplasm: Semifluid cytoplasm of muscle cells

sarcoplasmic reticulum: Network of tubules and sacs that plays an important role in muscle contraction and relaxation by releasing and storing calcium ions

segment: Line between waveforms; named by the waveform that precedes or follows it

semilunar valves: Valves shaped like half moons that separate the ventricles from the aorta and pulmonary artery

sensing: Ability of a pacemaker to recognize and respond to intrinsic electrical activity

septum: Partition

sick sinus syndrome: Term used to describe a sinus node dysfunction that may be manifested as severe sinus bradycardia, sinus arrest, sinus block, or bradycardia-tachycardia syndrome

sinoatrial node: Normal pacemaker of the heart that normally discharges at a rhythmic rate of 60 to 100 beats/min

sinus arrhythmia: Dysrhythmia originating in the sinoatrial node that occurs when the SA node discharges irregularly. Sinus arrhythmia is a normal phenomenon associated with the phases of respiration and changes in intrathoracic pressure

sinus bradycardia: Dysrhythmia originating in the sinoatrial node with a ventricular response of less than 60 beats/min

sinus tachycardia: Dysrhythmia originating in the sinoatrial node with a ventricular response between 101 to 180 beats/min

splanchnic: Pertaining to internal organs; visceral

ST segment: Portion of the ECG representing the end of ventricular depolarization (end of the R wave) and the beginning of ventricular repolarization (T wave)

stroke volume: Amount of blood ejected by either ventricle during one contraction; can be calculated as cardiac output divided by heart rate

subendocardial infarction: Myocardial infarction involving the endocardium and myocardium

subepicardial infarction: Myocardial infarction involving the myocardium and epicardium

sulcus: Groove

supraventricular: Originating from a site above the bundle branches, such as the sinoatrial node, atria, or AV junction

syncope: Fainting; usually resulting from cardiac or neurologic conditions including seizure disorders, vasodepressor syncope (the simple faint), and cardiac dysrhythmias

syncytium: Unit of combined cells

systole: Contraction of the heart (usually referring to ventricular contraction) during which blood is propelled into the pulmonary artery and aorta. When the term is used without reference to a specific chamber of the heart, the term implies ventricular systole

tachycardia: Heart rate greater than 100 beats/min (tachy = fast)

threshold: Membrane potential at which the cell membrane will depolarize and generate an action potential

TKO: Abbreviation meaning "to keep open;" also known as KVO, "keep the vein open"

torsades de pointes (TdP): Type of polymorphic VT associated with a prolonged QT interval. The QRS changes in shape, amplitude, and width and appears to "twist" around the isoelectric line, resembling a spindle

transmural infarction: Myocardial infarction in which the entire thickness of the ventricular wall (endocardium to epicardium) is involved

trifascicular block: Block in the three primary divisions of the bundle branches (i.e., right bundle branch, left anterior fascicle, and left posterior fascicle)

trigeminy: Dysrhythmia in which every third beat is a premature ectopic beat

unipolar lead: Lead that consists of a single positive electrode and a reference point; a pacing lead with a single electrical pole at the distal tip of the pacing lead (negative pole) through which the stimulating pulse is delivered. In a permanent pacemaker with a unipolar lead, the positive pole is the pulse generator case

VA interval: In dual-chamber pacing, the interval between a sensed or ventricular-paced event and the next atrial-paced event

VV interval: Interval between two ventricular-paced events

V wave: Ventricular-paced event; the ventricular stimulus or the point in the intrinsic ventricular depolarization (R wave) during which ventricular sensing occurs

vagal maneuver: Methods used to stimulate the vagus nerve in an attempt to slow conduction through the AV node, resulting in slowing of the heart rate

vector: Quantity having direction and magnitude, usually depicted by a straight arrow whose length represents magnitude and whose head represents direction

venous return: Amount of blood flowing into the right atrium each minute from the systemic circulation

ventricle: Either of the two lower chambers of the heart

ventricular pacing: Pacing system with a lead attached in the right ventricle

ventricular tachycardia (VT): Dysrhythmia originating in the ventricles with a ventricular response greater than 100 beats/min

wandering atrial pacemaker (multiformed atrial rhythm): Cardiac dysrhythmia that occurs because of impulses originating from various sites, including the sinoatrial node, the atria, and/or the AV junction. Requires at least three different P waves, seen in the same lead, for proper diagnosis

waveform: Movement away from the baseline in either a positive or negative direction

Wolff-Parkinson-White syndrome: Type of preexcitation syndrome characterized by a slurred upstroke of the QRS complex (delta wave) and wide QRS

Credits

CHAPTER 1

Figures 1-1, 1-2, 1-3: Thibodeau G, Patton K: *Anatomy and physiology,* ed 4, St Louis, 1999, Mosby.

Figure 1-4: *Managing major diseases: cardiac disorders,* vol 2, ed 2, St Louis, 1999, Mosby.

Figure 1-5: Thibodeau G, Patton K: *Anatomy and physiology,* ed 4, St Louis, 1999, Mosby.

Figure 1-6: Herlihy B, Maebius N: *The human body in health and illness,* Philadelphia, 2000, WB Saunders.

Figure 1-7: Cannobio M: *Cardiovascular disorders, Mosby's clinical nursing series,* St Louis, 1990, Mosby.

Figure 1-8: Thibodeau G, Patton K: *Anatomy and physiology,* ed 4, St Louis, 1999, Mosby.

CHAPTER 2

Figure 2-1: Thibodeau G, Patton K: *Anatomy and physiology,* ed 4, St Louis, 1999, Mosby.

Figures 2-2, 2-3, 2-4: Herlihy B, Maebius N: *The human body in health and illness,* Philadelphia, 2000, WB Saunders.

Figure 2-5: Crawford M, Spence M: *Commonsense approach to coronary care,* ed 6, St Louis, 1995, Mosby.

Figure 2-6: Guyton A, Hall J: *Textbook of medical physiology,* ed 9, Philadelphia, 1996, WB Saunders.

Figure 2-7: Marriot H, Conover M: *Advanced concepts in arrhythmias,* ed 3, St Louis, 1998, Mosby.

Figure 2-8: Phalen T: *The 12-lead ECG in acute myocardial infarction,* St Louis, 1996, Mosby.

Figures 2-9, 2-10, 2-11: Thelan L, Urden L, Lough M, et al: *Critical care nursing: diagnosis and management,* ed 2, St Louis, 1998, Mosby.

Figure 2-12: Clochesy J, Breu C, Cardin S, et al: *Critical care nursing,* ed 2, Philadelphia, 1996, WB Saunders.

Figure 2-13: Lounsbury P, Frye S: *Cardiac rhythm disorders,* ed 2, St Louis, 1992, Mosby.

Figures 2-15, 2-16, 2-19: Goldberger A: *Clinical electrocardiography: a simplified approach,* ed 6, St Louis, 1999, Mosby.

Figure 2-20: Thelan L, Urden L, Lough M, et al: *Critical care nursing: diagnosis and management,* ed 2, St Louis, 1998, Mosby.

Figure 2-22: Goldberger A: *Clinical electrocardiography: a simplified approach,* ed 6, St Louis, 1999, Mosby.

Figure 2-23: Chou T: *Electrocardiography in clinical practice: adult and pediatric,* ed 4, Philadelphia, 1996, WB Saunders.

Figures 2-24, 2-25: Thibodeau G, Patton K: *Anatomy and physiology,* ed 4, St Louis, 1999, Mosby.

Figures 2-26, 2-27, 2-28: Sanders M: *Mosby's paramedic textbook,* St Louis, 1994, Mosby.

CHAPTER 4

Figure 4-2: Kinney M, Packa D, Andreoli K, et al: *Andreoli's comprehensive cardiac care,* ed 8, St Louis, 1995, Mosby.

Figure 4-4: Goldberger A: *Clinical electrocardiography: a simplified approach,* ed 6, St Louis, 1999, Mosby.

Figure 4-6: Thelan L, Urden L, Lough M, et al: *Critical care nursing: diagnosis and management,* ed 2, St Louis, 1998, Mosby.

Figure 4-8: Crawford M, Spence M: *Commonsense approach to coronary care,* ed 6, St Louis, 1995, Mosby.

Figure 4-9: Chou T: *Electrocardiography in clinical practice: adult and pediatric,* ed 4, Philadelphia, 1996, WB Saunders.

Figure 4-12: Goldberger A: *Clinical electrocardiography: a simplified approach,* ed 6, St Louis, 1999, Mosby.

CHAPTER 6

Figure 6-6: Chou T: *Electrocardiography in clinical practice: adult and pediatric* ed 4, Philadelphia, 1996, WB Saunders.

CHAPTER 9

Figure 9-1: Thelan L, Urden L, Lough M, et al: *Critical care nursing: diagnosis and management,* ed 2, St Louis, 1998, Mosby.
Figure 9-2: Phalen T: *The 12-lead ECG in acute myocardial infarction,* St Louis, 1996, Mosby.
Figure 9-3: Goldberger A: *Clinical electrocardiography: a simplified approach,* ed 6, St Louis, 1999, Mosby.
Figures 9-4, 9-5: Phalen T: *The 12-lead ECG in acute myocardial infarction,* St Louis, 1996, Mosby.
Figure 9-6: Kinney M, Packa D, Andreoli K, et al: *Andreoli's comprehensive cardiac care,* ed 8, St Louis, 1995, Mosby.
Figure 9-7: Phalen T: *The 12-lead ECG in acute myocardial infarction,* St Louis, 1996, Mosby.

Index

WWW.Cardiomonitor.com

WWW.medi-smart.com/tutorial site
www.learnwell.org/ekg htm

www.ecglibrary.com

www.aafp.org/online/en/home/
www.emergeyekg.compurtic
www.

2-6-03   Glucometer
Coleen Bartels   Class
4/10-532-4527
    Beeper 18u

QRS .12 >= B B B
PRI >.2 Q = 1° Blk

ULTRA Vitamits

Soy Nuts
ces.com/ekghtm...
www.learnwell.org/ekg.htm